TRADITIONAL MEDICINE IN AFRICA

COVER: The cover photograph shows the Kikuyu medicineman's kit *mũano* containing the diagnostic, surgical and therapeutic paraphernalia. The medicineman (*mũndũ mũgo*) used the kit for both managing illness and performing magic (see Kikuyu Traditional Medicine – Chapter 11). The big gourd *kĩnya kĩa mbogo* contains stone pebbles, marbles, hair, flesh, etc. used in diagnosis; the two small gourds contain *ira*, a powdery material, used in surgical operations; the 'stirrer', made of animal vertebrae, used to stir concoctions; and the knife used in surgery. (PHOTO BY BARRACK MULUKA. Courtesy of the Institute of African Studies.)

TRADITIONAL MEDICINE IN AFRICA

Edited by

Isaac Sindiga

Chacha Nyaigotti-Chacha

and

Mary Peter Kanunah

East African Educational Publishers Ltd
NAIROBI

Published by
East African Educational Publishers Ltd
Brick Court
Mpaka Road/Woodvale Grove
Westlands
P. O. Box 45314
Nairobi

First published 1995

ISBN 9966 - 46 - 548 - 0

Typeset by
Ramani Cartographic Services
P. O. Box 38950
Nairobi

Printed by,
English Press Ltd.,
Enterprise Road,
P.O. Box 30127, Nairobi.

Contents

Preface
List of contributors
List of Figures
List of Tables

Chapter

1	Traditional Medicine in Africa: An Introduction —*Isaac Sindiga*	1
2	African Ethnomedicine and Other Medical Systems —*Isaac Sindiga*	16
3	A Case for Traditional Medicine in Official Health Services— *David O. Nyamwaya*	30
4	Confidence in Traditional Healers— *Richard M. Swiderski*	40
5	Ethnomedical Practice in Kenya: The Case of Karati Rural Service Centre —*Jack K. Githae*	55
6	Managing Illness Among the Luo—*Isaac Sindiga*	64
7	Ethnomedical Remedies and Therapies in Maternal and Child Health Among the Rural Luo —*Evelynes Agot Kawango*	80
8	Maasai Traditional Medicine —*Isaac Sindiga*	94
9	Gusii Traditional Medicine —*Isaac Sindiga*	108

10 Traditional Medicine Among the Abaluyia —*Simiyu Wandibba* 117

11 Kikuyu Traditional Medicine—*I. Sindiga, M. P. Kanunah E. M. Aseka and G. W. Kiriga* 129

12 The Role of Traditional Medicine in a Rural Environment—*S. R. Baquar* 140

13 Management of Medicinal Plant Resources in Nyanza —*E. A. O. Obado and J. E. Odera* 153

14 Drug Research Priorities in Kenya with Special Emphasis on Traditional Medicine —*W. M. Kofi-Tsekpo* 168

15 The Future of Traditional Medicine in Africa — *I. Sindiga, M. P. Kanunah, C. Nyaigotti-Chacha and E. S. Mwangola* 175

Appendix A: Application for the Registration of Traditional Medical Practitioners 185

Appendix B: Application Form for the Registration of Traditional Medicines 187

Index 193

Dedicated with great love

To Brian Ayaga Sindiga. May you grow to cherish the heritage of your people.

And

To all indigenous health workers whose silent contribution to humanity is much appreciated.

Preface

The idea of this book goes back to a day in August 1991. While on a visit to the offices of the International Development Research Centre (IDRC) in Nairobi, one of us appraised Dr. Firoze Manji, then a representative of the Health Sciences Division (now at the Aga Khan Foundation in London), on his project on 'Ethnomedicine and Health Care in Kenya' which was reaching completion, and discussed his plans for a workshop on 'Traditional Medicine, Its Practice and the Law in Kenya'. Dr. Manji gave him the go-ahead to prepare a proposal and submit it to IDRC for possible funding. The workshop was subsequently held at the Lake Bogoria Hotel between November 4th and 7th, 1992.

The motivation for the workshop was that the majority of Kenyans – rural and urban, illiterate and literate, spanning a myriad ethnic and religious affiliations, utilize traditional medicine at one time or the other. For many rural Kenyans, modern health care is both inaccessible and unavailable, and hence use traditional medicine as a matter of course. Kenya's quest to attain "health for all by the year 2000" led to a reorientation towards the primary health care approach which calls for the incorporation of traditional medicine and its practitioners in official health care delivery.* Whereas some research has been undertaken on various aspects of indigenous medical systems, more work is required on the role, use and organization of traditional medicine.

Another problem of traditional medicine is its uncertain legal position in the country's statute books. Yet, the practice of traditional medicine requires legal protection if it has to contribute meaningfully in the primary health care programme.

The Lake Bogoria Workshop, believed to be the first national gathering of its kind ever, brought together various workers in the ethnomedical field to review

---

* Bennett, F. J. and J. Maneno, (eds). *National Guidelines for the Implementation of Primary Health Care in Kenya.* Nairobi: Ministry of Health the Non-Governmental Health Organizations of Kenya, World Health Organization and UNICEF, 1986), Chapter 3.

the practice of traditional medicine in Kenya. (The detailed workshop objectives can be pursued elsewhere).* Here, we provide only a summary:

- To explore traditional medicine, its practice and organization;
- To review the utilization of traditional medicine;
- To examine the legal aspects of traditional medicinal practice including criminal and civil liability, and protection under the law;
- To sensitize policy makers and scholars about previous and ongoing research in traditional medicine; and,
- To provide recommendations to guide future policy, legislation and research on traditional medicine.

These objectives were met to varying degrees of success judging by the workshop product.

Among the stated objectives of the Lake Bogoria Workshop was to publish the proceedings for reference and to offer the deliberations to the wider academy. At the conclusion of the workshop, a small team, comprising the editors and Emma Mwangola, stayed an extra day to deliberate on the proceedings of the previous three days. This enabled Prof. Nyaigotti-Chacha to participate as co-editor. We decided that rather than publish the entire proceedings, a number of papers from the workshop be selected for this book. This would allow us to exclude papers which did not meet project objectives and those which did not exhibit substantial scholarship. Another criterion for selection was the comments made on the papers during the workshop.

Having deliberated on the proceedings, the next step was to invite critical commentary from a number of scholars to guide the authors during revision and to aid the editorial process. We are grateful to Dr. W. M. Kofi-Tsekpo, Prof. P. K. Ndalut and the editors for returning their comments in record time.

Henry Chakava of the East African Educational Publishers Ltd showed interest in this project right from its initiation. He read an earlier draft of the manuscript and obtained an independent anonymous reviewer to provide opinion on the work. Their comments were useful in the preparation of this book.

The initial title of this work was 'Traditional Medicine in Kenya'. This was aimed at reflecting the mandate of the original manuscript. The current title

---

* Sindiga, I. (ed.) *Traditional Medicine: Its Practice and the Law in Kenya.* Proceedings of the National Workshop at the Lake Bogoria Hotel, 4-7 November, 1992 (Eldoret: Moi University, 1993).

emerged after a major review whereby several new chapters, not originally presented at the workshop, were added to improve the conceptual foundations of the work and case study coverage.

We did not provide a strict structure by which the chapters would be written. Each contributor had considerable latitude in selecting his/her own format. This inevitably led to some overlaps which were, however, considerably reduced during the editorial process. The result is readable and compelling scholarship on the subject.

The bulk of the editorial work was done at Moi University. Mary Kanunah performed countless tasks and worked into the Christmas of 1992 to produce the first draft. She selflessly helped improve the quality of the book in several ways—proof reading, verifying bibliographic entries and co-authoring two chapters. We are grateful to Jane Wangusi who tirelessly helped in many ways which included forwarding mail, typing and photocopying, despite her family responsibilities. Thanks also to Alice Orembo for typing many versions of the manuscript and to Juliet Rop for typing the final draft.

We acknowledge support from various organisations, namely, the International Development Research Centre and Moi University for financial support in respect of the Lake Bogoria workshop. Isaac Sindiga is grateful for the support accorded him by IDRC and the Rockefeller Foundation. His contributions in this book, being products of work he undertook between 1989 and 1993, were funded by both organizations.

Finally, we would be remiss not to acknowledge the cooperation of the various contributors in this volume who are medical people, anthropologists, historians, educationists, botanists, foresters and geographers. This is thus a multidisciplinary piece of work which clearly defines the problem of practising traditional medicine in Africa. The common purpose is to contribute towards sensitizing policy makers and the academic community about the underdevelopment of traditional medicine.

It is our hope that clinicians, medical students, health planners, social scientists and policy makers will find the information in this volume invaluable. This will justify the many hours spent in the preparation of *Traditional Medicine in Africa.*

ISAAC SINDIGA
CHACHA NYAIGOTTI-CHACHA
MARY P. KANUNAH
March 1995

Editorial Note: There are some differences in Luo terminologies in some chapters of this book. This is attributed to differences in language between Siaya and South Nyanza regions where the respective studies were carried out

List of Contributors

Eric M. ASEKA is Senior Lecturer and Chairman, Department of History, Kenyatta University.

S.R. BAQUAR was formerly Professor and Head, Department of Botany, Moi University. He has done extensive research on traditional medicinal herbs in Pakistan and Kenya.

Jack K. GITHAE is a traditional medical practitioner and proprietor of Karati Herbal Clinics based at Naivasha, Kenya.

Mary P. KANUNAH is a geographer currently teaching in the Department of Tourism, Moi University. She is co-editor of this book.

Evelynes Agot KAWANGO is a lecturer in geography at Moi University. She is a registered D. Phil student at the University researching in medical geography.

Gladys W. KIRIGA is a lecturer in history at the Laikipia College Campus, Egerton University.

W. M. KOFI-TSEKPO is Chief Research Officer and Director, Traditional Medicines and Drugs Research Centre, Kenya Medical Research Institute, Nairobi.

Emma S. MWANGOLA is lecturer, Department of Languages and Linguistics, Egerton University.

Chacha NYAIGOTTI-CHACHA is Principal, Kisii College Campus and Associate Professor of Languages and Linguistics at Egerton University. He is a co-editor (with Isaac Sindiga and Mary P. Kanunah) of this volume.

David O. NYAMWAYA is a medical anthropologist and Director of the Health Behaviour and Education Department at the African Medical and Research Foundation in Nairobi. He has done extensive research on traditional medicine in Kenya.

E. A. Ochieng, OBADO is Lecturer, Department of Forestry, Moi University.

J. A. ODERA is the Director, Kenya Forestry Research Institute.

Isaac SINDIGA is Associate Professor of Geography and Head, Department of Tourism, Moi University. He is co-editor of this volume and has done detailed field research on the role of ethnomedicine in health care in Kenya.

Richard M. SWIDERSKI was formerly Senior Lecturer, Department of Anthropology, Moi University.

Simiyu WANDIBBA is the Director, Institute of African Studies, University of Nairobi.

List of Acronyms

CBHC	Community based health care
CIKARD	Centre for Indigenous Knowledge for Agriculture and Rural Development
CIRAN	Centre for International Research and Advisory Networks
CMR	Child mortality rate
FAO	Food and Agriculture Organization
IDRC	International Development Research Centre
KEFRI	Kenya Forestry Research Institute
KEMRI	Kenya Medical Research Institute
KRSC	Karati Rural Service Centre
LEAD	Leiden Ethnosystems and Development Programme
MCH	Maternal child health
NCST	National Council for Science and Technology
PHC	Primary health care
TBA	Traditional birth attendant
UNEP	United Nations Environemntal Programme
UNICEF	United Nations Children's Fund
USAID	United States Agency for International Development
WHA	World Health Assembly
WHO	World Health Organization
GNP	Gross National Product

List of Figures

		Page
8.1	Stages in the development of a Maasai medicineman	99
8.2	Nested hierarchy of Maasai medicinemen	100

List of Tables

		Page
1.1	Major ethnomedical systems	3
1.2	Percentage distribution of household members receiving non-institution treatment by province	6
5.1	KRSC patient attendance, 1984-90	57
5.2	Origin of patients to KRSC	58
5.3	Percentage contribution of various plant parts to herbal medicine at K.R.S.C.	60
6.1	Major categories of Luo traditional healers	69
6.2	Basic characteristics of consumers of traditional medicines in South Nyanza	74
8.1	Some herbal medicines and drugs used by the Maasai	96
8.2	Major categories of Maasai traditional healers	98
8.3	Aggregate numbers of traditional healers in Narok	103
9.1	Major categories of Gusii traditional healers	112
11.1	Causes of ill health among the pre-colonial Kikuyu	131
13.1	Families and traditional healers visited in Nyanza Province	155
13.2	Some common medicinal plant species marketed in Kisumu town but harvested from outside the Province	159
13.3	Some important species harvested by uprooting the whole plant	160
13.4	Source/origin of medicinal plants by district	161
13.5	Valuable forest timber species found in Kenyan forests partially or fully ring-barked for herbal medicines	162
13.6	Some tree species in Nyanza found in farms partially or fully ring-barked species for herbal medicines	163
15.1	Major characteristics of allopathic and ethnomedical practices	180

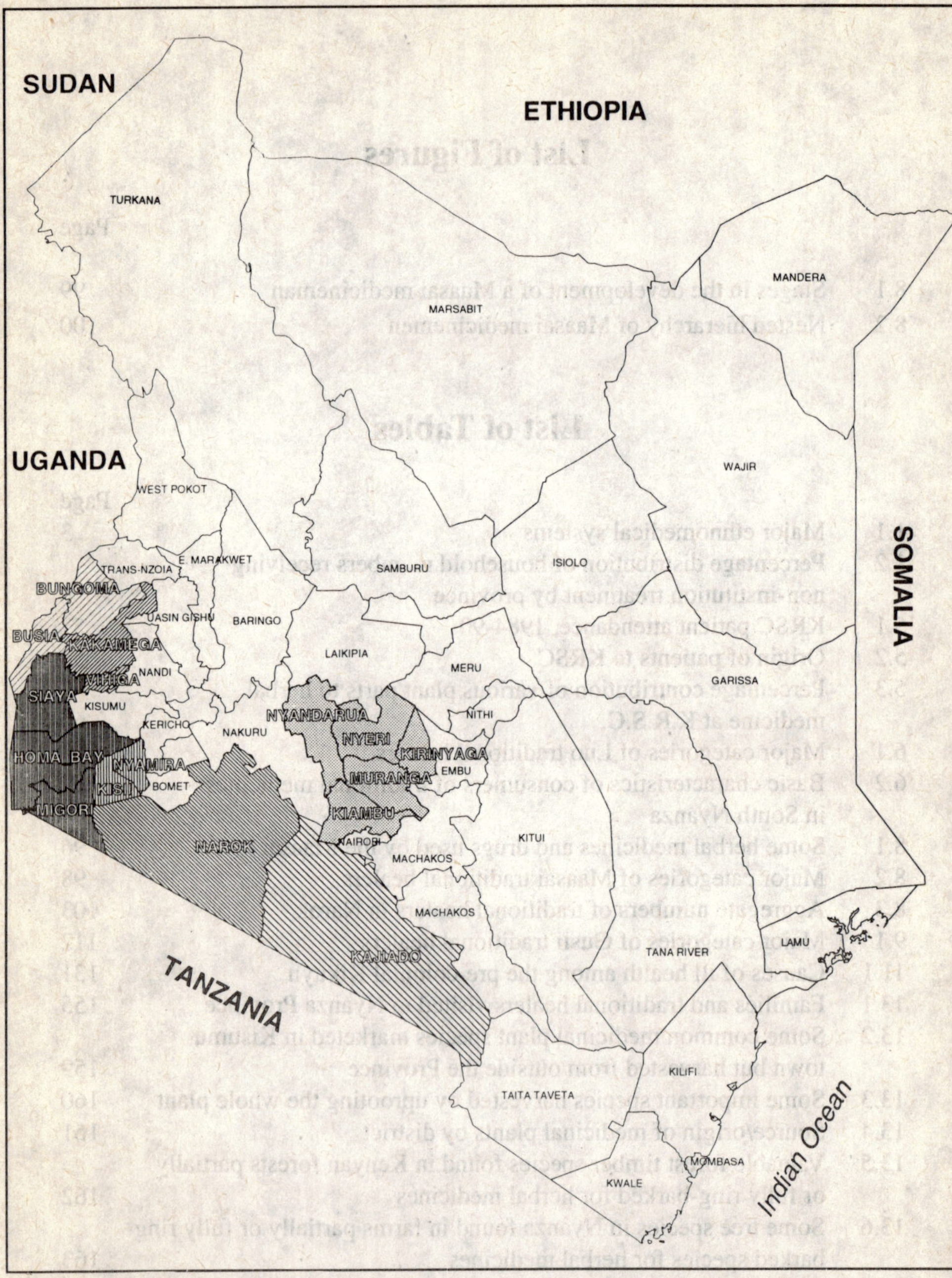

Map of Kenya: The shaded areas show regions referred to by the authors

Chapter 1

TRADITIONAL MEDICINE IN AFRICA An Introduction

Isaac Sindiga

The Case for Traditional Medicine

For more than two decades now the World Health Organization (WHO) has encouraged the use of traditional medicine, especially in the developing countries by promoting the incorporation of its useful elements into national health care systems (Akerele, 1987). In particular, the immense human resources in traditional medicine could be utilized in official health care.

Part of the reason for using traditional medicine is that the biomedical (or Western system of medicine), which is popularized by governments, cannot cope with current morbidity and mortality rates. Whereas it is difficult to make generalizations about health conditions in the Third World (as these vary from one region to another and even within individual countries), overall, life expectancy at birth is low. Tropical Africa records a life expectancy of 51 years (Feachem, Jamison and Bos, 1991). Mortality rate is high especially for children below five years of age — some 14.5 million children die every year in developing countries (Earickson, et. al., 1989), while 10 per cent of all births end up in death by the first birthday and 20 per cent by the fifth birthday (Caldwell, 1991: 227). Maternal deaths are high as well. According to WHO data, a woman in tropical Africa has a "one in 21 chance of dying of pregnancy-related causes during her reproductive life, compared with a one in 54 chance in Asia, and one in 2,089 in Europe" (Graham, 1991).

The high morbidity rate in Africa is as a result of parasitic infectious diseases. Diseases such as malaria, schistosomiasis and trypanosomiasis are endemic in many parts and thereby affect labour productivity, especially in respect of agriculture. The specific causes of morbidity and mortality are respiratory infections (e.g. pneumonia, tuberculosis and whooping cough) and water-borne diseases (e.g. dysentery, typhoid and cholera). These diseases are related to poor housing with little ventilation as well as sanitation — clean water supplies are often unavailable and waste disposal is a problem. For instance, with regard to human waste, many people do not have pit latrines and thus help themselves in the bush. This waste is often collected by rain water and taken to rivers where people water their livestock and also fetch water for domestic use.

Fertility is equally high and is related to the high mortality rate especially among infants and children. Yet, the primary cause of mortality among children under five years is malnutrition which is widespread in Africa (Ofosu–Amaah, 1991); per capita food productivity has remarkably declined over the past four decades (World Bank, 1989). This has been caused by debilitating droughts, floods, inability to raise production due to non-adoption of innovations (partly due to high cost), and strife (which has occurred in almost every corner of the continent).

These health problems notwithstanding, the level of health services remain very low in the developing countries (Feachem and Jamison, 1991; World Bank, 1989). Yet, the large public and private health expenditures in most of the countries, averaging between six and 10 per cent of the GNP have not taken health services close to the people, so that health care has remained inaccessible to the majority of the population.

The inadequacy of health services could partly be explained by historical emphasis on costly, hospital-based curative care which put premium on expensive technology and the meeting of international health standards whilst ignoring local disease problems. Even where health facilities exist, these suffer from shortage of trained health workers, inadequate supplies and poor management, all translating into non-availability of services (Pillsbury, 1979; World Bank, 1980). Again, some of the services are not socially acceptable as they largely ignore the participation of local communities.

By mid-1970s it had become clear that modern health care was getting more and more remote from the majority of the population in the rural areas. Moreover, tropical Africa's rapid population growth rate (averaging an annual 3%) ate into whatever gains were achieved in expanding medical services. Therefore, the solution to the accessibility problem did not seem to lie in building more and more facilities; it could be improved by a shift in policy, from curative care to preventive and promotive services.

From 1975, UNICEF and WHO began to emphasize the primary health care (PHC) approach which would utilize local human and material support available in a community to provide the underserved population (Akerele, 1987; Golladay and Liese, 1980). This approach, based on the utilization of a community's local resources, meant the inclusion of traditional medical practitioners. The programme involved immunization, maternal and child health, family planning, nutrition, curative services, health education, environmental health (clean water supply, sanitation etc), and early diagnosis and treatment of diseases.

The approach (PHC) was adopted at the 1978 Alma Ata International Conference on Primary Health Care where 134 countries and 64 United Nations agencies were represented. The Conference declared health a universal human right and issued a declaration urging governments to provide accessible, affordable and socially relevant health care to each individual (Golladay and Liese, 1980). The goal of this approach was "Health for All By 2000".

Traditional Medicine in Primary Health Care

As noted earlier, the primary health care approach calls specifically for the use of traditional medicine — both the pharmacopoeia and practitioners. Towards this end, WHO encourages the incorporation of useful elements of traditional medicine into national health care systems (Akerele, 1987).

Table 1.1: Major ethnomedical systems

System	Remarks
Ayurveda	Hindu medicine. Practised by Indian immigrants elsewhere. Used in Nepal as well.
Yoga	Used in India and wherever Indian immigrants have settled.
Unani	Arabic medicine. Now used in South Asia.
Siddha	Used in South India.
Chinese	Used in mainland China and among the Chinese populations elsewhere. Includes Han medicine and various systems practised by minorities such as Dai, Mongolian, Tibetan and Uighur.
African traditional	Each of Africa's multiplicity of communities has its own medical system. Disease aetiologies and treatment procedures tend to be similar.
Homeopathy, Chiropractic & acupuncture	Used as alternative therapies in developed countries. Acupuncture is Chinese in origin.

The history of the use of traditional medicine with WHO goes back to 1977 when the World Health Assembly (WHA) drew attention to the potential of traditional medicine, especially its human power reserve in national health care systems, urging member countries to utilize traditional medicines (Akerele, 1987; Nakajima, 1987). Then in 1978, it highlighted the crucial role of medicinal herbs in the health care systems of many developing countries. This was reinforced by the Alma Ata Conference which recommended that governments give priority to utilizing traditional medicines in national drug policies and regulations (Akerele, 1987). These resolutions and recommendations regarding traditional medicine were reaffirmed at the 40th World Health Assembly held in May, 1987 (Nakajima, 1987).

Perhaps Pillsbury (1979) best encapsulated the necessity for utilizing indigenous medical practitioners in health care delivery when she captured the essence of using traditional medicine. She argued that if the majority of rural populations in developing countries have to be reached by some form of official health care, then efforts have to be made to use local resources. She further noted that large numbers of the rural people do not always utilize existing official health care services — most of them are suspicious of Western medicine partly because it does not tolerate local beliefs and behaviour related to health matters and is partly the reason why some 90 per cent of the rural population seeks health care in traditional medicine (Pillsbury, 1979, see Table 1.1.). In Zimbabwe, traditional healers are consulted on a large variety of health problems (McIvor, 1989) and so is the case in Zambia (Twumasi, 1984). It is estimated that over 75 per cent of the rural population in Africa seeks health care among traditional healers (Ampofo and Johnson–Romauld, 1978). Therefore, throughout tropical Africa, traditional medicine is thriving. From West Africa to Central Africa, and Eastern Africa to Southern Africa, traditional medicine is being evaluated with a view to instituting its participation in the national health care systems (Pillsbury, 1982; Warren, 1988). This follows the practice where certain countries in Asia such as Sri Lanka, India, China, Bhutan, Nepal and Vietnam have integrated ethnomedicine with modern medicine in official health care (WHO, 1985; Guo–Bin, 1987).

Apparently, the rudimentary and strained network of modern health facilities in developing countries, particularly those of tropical Africa, is coming under great pressure especially with the emergence of the AIDS pandemic whose rapid rate of expansion spells a higher infant and child mortality and hence foreshadows the region's future (Preble, 1990). Already, the infant and child mortality in tropical Africa is high and this problem is not solved by running an under-developed health care service. Traditional medicine is advocated for a number of reasons:

(1) It is an integral part of every culture developed over many years. Thus, it is effective in curing certain cultural health problems.

(2) It is socially acceptable.
(3) It has the widest spatial coverage; each community has its own healers. It is thus the surest way of moving towards attaining health for all by the turn of the century.
(4) It is holistic in approach. It views disease and illness to be disequilibrium of social groups with the total environment (See Chapter 2).
(5) It is efficacious.
(6) Traditional healers charge affordable fees (WHO, 1978; Pillsbury, 1979; Phillips, 1985).

The compelling reason, however, is its ability to meet "the four criteria of accessibility, availability, acceptability and dependability" (Nchinda, 1976:134). This is the *raison d'etre* for evaluating and recognizing traditional medicine with a view to improving "its efficacy, safety, availability, and wider application at low cost" (World Bank, 1980). But first, research is required "to discover more about the role of traditional medical practitioners in their communities" as the initial step towards formulating effective policies regarding their role in PHC (WHO, 1985:15).

Traditional Medicine in Kenya

Kenya's modern health facilities are spatially inequitable and favour urban areas where only about 15 per cent of the country's 25 million population lives. Some 57 per cent of the households in Kenya must travel more than 4 kilometres to the nearest health facility; only 30 per cent of the population lives within 2 kilometres of a health facility (Bennett and Maneno, 1986). Even among the urban set-up, only the primate towns of Nairobi and Mombasa enjoy accessible and available health care. Country-wide, the ratios of health centre to population vary from 1:200,000 to 1:50,000, a far cry from the government target of 1:20,000 and less. The ratio of doctors to the population has shown little improvement since independence (in 1963) partly because of the rapid population growth rate – the population grew at 3 per cent per year in the 1960s and peaked at 4 per cent in the 1970s and 1980s. In addition, some 75 per cent of Kenya's health workers live and work in the major urban centres.

Besides, there are great regional disparities in the distribution of health facilities so that the majority of the rural population in many districts has no access to modern health care. A decade ago, only about 30 per cent of the population in South Nyanza District lived close enough to modern health facilities (Kenya, 1984). Most of the rural population in Turkana District had no contact with modern medicine either due to reliance on traditional therapies or due to the fact that modern health facilities were beyond reach in terms of distance, awareness and finance (Kenya, 1980). This situation has not changed much.

Even where health facilities exist, medical service is not always available. Many facilities suffer from inadequate personnel, shortage of drugs, transport problems, lack of water, delays in repairs and even lack of stationery. Other problems include financial constraints to expand the services, low community participation, physical inaccessibility and remoteness (especially in the semi-arid and arid areas of the country), congestion (frequently there is more than 100% bed occupancy) and the high cost of curative care. The inability to reach modern health facilities is a major reason as to why most rural Kenyans look up to traditional medicine for the treatment of various ailments (Good, 1987; Good and Kimani, 1980). Moreover, 80 per cent of all births in the country are conducted at home by traditional birth attendants rather than by midwives in maternity hospital wards (Chief Nursing Officer, 1991: iii).

However, this physical and economic inaccessibility of modern medicine explains only a part of the Kenyans' behaviour in seeking treatment in traditional medicine. The evidence is unmitigated that Kenyans, just like people in other African countries, may not seek Western medicine even when this is accessible

Table 1.2: Percentage distribution of household members in Kenya receiving non-institutional treatment by province

	Coast	Eastern	Central	R. Valley	Nyanza	Western	National figures
Shop	74.7	67.0	35.7	46.0	56.3	57.6	57.6
Self Medication	2.4	20.1	60.0	42.5	19.8	21.9	25.6
Traditional Medical practitioners	22.3	11.6	1.2	10.3	16.7	16.9	13.9
Others	0.6	1.3	3.1	1.2	7.2	3.6	2.9
Totals	100.0	100.0	100.0	100.0	100.0	100.0	100.0

SOURCE: Republic of Kenya, *The Integrated Rural Surveys 1976-79* (Nairobi: Central Bureau of Statistics, 1982), p. 62.

(see Chapter 2) owing to social, psychological or cultural reasons (Mayer, 1982; Nchinda, 1976; Katz and Kimani, 1982; Good and Kimani, 1980; Pillsbury, 1979). In certain instances, people utilize both traditional and modern medicine simultaneously (see Chapter 6).

Kenyans seek therapy from a variety of sources (Chapter 3). Research conducted some two decades ago found that 17 per cent of 2.6 million people who sought non-licensed, non-institutional treatment in traditional medicine, obtained it from traditional healers (Table 1.2). The figure may be much larger as people are unwilling to admit openly that they consult with traditional healers. Good (1980) found that in the sprawling Mathare slum of Nairobi, there was one traditional healer to a population of 847. This is relatively high patronage.

In spite of the prominent role that traditional medicine plays in health care in Kenya, it is the least understood of all medical systems. Kenya has no legislation governing the production and registration of traditional medicines some of which have been proven to be effective with regard to several ailments (see Chapter 14). As a result, the medicines are currently being harvested and exported without restriction.

Notwithstanding official acknowledgment that traditional medicine is "an important part of life of the people in the rural areas" (Kenya, 1979: 136; Kenya, 1989:244), policy makers and biomedical practitioners frequently dismiss it. As a result, little is known about it, its practice and how it is organized.

Both modern and traditional medicine have co-existed as parallel systems with little coordination between them. In the 1979-1983 Development Plan, the government called for research "to evaluate the role and functions and to determine the extent of the need for traditional medicine" (Kenya, 1979:136). Much of the research into traditional medicine has, however, centred on the medicinal value and efficacy of the herbs and other pharmacopoeia (Kokwaro, 1976) and such is the research carried out at the Kenya Medical Research Institute (KEMRI) and the Traditional Medicines Unit of the Department of Pharmacy, University of Nairobi. Thus, government policy appears to encourage research in traditional medicines in order to provide scientific basis for drugs (Kenya, 1994:235).

It is the intent of this book to contribute data on many aspects of traditional medicine and its role in health care. The book is a first step towards evaluating how the traditional medical systems can contribute towards primary health care. This work meets an already set national objective, namely "to determine the importance and relevance of traditional medicine with regard to both its substantive aspects and its potential link with government institutions" (Kenya, 1979:136). The commitment to adopt appropriate traditional diagnostic, therapeutic and rehabilitative control technologies so as to become part of

Kenya's formal medical research and PHC follows Thairu's (1975) plea and was reiterated in the 1989-1993 National Development Plan (Kenya, 1989).

The Organization of the Book

This book comprises a collection of essays based on lessons and analysis of various aspects of traditional medicine in Africa. Ultimately it defines the problem of practising traditional medicine and, by extension, the malady of Africa's health systems.

Scope

Reading through these essays, a number of salient points come out. The major issues that stand out in almost all the chapters are that:

- traditional medicine is widely used.
- traditional medicines are effective.
- medicinal herbs are threatened by population pressures, destruction by indiscriminate harvesting and foreign export.
- traditional medicine requires to be protected, enhanced and developed. But first, an enabling environment, beginning with specific legislation recognizing traditional medicine, is required.
- there is need for more research institutions to undertake chemical analysis of traditional drugs.

The book does not cover all the areas of the subjects, rather, it is an effort to highlight the main themes of this complex, interdisciplinary and multidisciplinary area of traditional medicine. It is expected that this book will spur interest and research into this important aspect of the lives of many Africans.

Other issues raised in this book relate to personnel in traditional medicine. These are; lack of uniform training of traditional medical practitioners and lack of a clearly defined organizational framework within which traditional healers operate.

These essays have been prepared by a multidisciplinary team of experts which include clinicians, botanists, traditional medical practitioners, educationists, anthropologists, historians, foresters and geographers.

Presentation of the essays

The style and presentation of the essays are inevitably varied. However, one thing stands out about all the essays; the cases are original. Most chapters in this book are based on painstaking field research and observations. There are chapters that consist of critical reviews of the subject while others are significant for their blending of theory and empirical observations and yet others are of applied significance and offer specific recommendations for further action. The following is a brief overview of each of the essays:

Chapter 2 sets out the conceptual foundations of African ethnomedicine as it relates to other medical systems (including biomedicine or the so-called modern medical system). The basis, philosophy and characteristics of African ethnomedical systems are outlined. This is a prelude to the discussion on the possibilities of cooperation among the various medical systems within communities where medical pluralism exists. At the end of the discussion, the author considers how the disciplinary bounds of medical geography could provide a fruitful framework for research in traditional medicine.

In *Chapter 3*, D. O. Nyamwaya provides an overview of traditional medicine in Kenya. While acknowledging Kenya's rural medical landscapes, he discusses the interaction of indigenous and cosmopolitan medicine with regard to health seeking behaviour. The interaction may be sequential, zig-zag, supplementary, complementary or competitive. He decries the unregulated mushrooming of traditional medical practitioners with several negative effects including delayed referral, malpractice, misuse of drugs and persistence of negative attitudes to traditional medicine. He regrets the fact that there is hardly any technical support to traditional medicine and provides a proposal for improving traditional medicine as a component of official health care.

In *Chapter 4*, Richard Swiderski uses a model and selected cases to discuss public confidence in traditional healers — most urban traditional healers are innovating by adopting certain biomedical procedures while retaining the more personal and local aspects of traditional medicine. He notes that this is an effort to gain the confidence of an urbanizing clientele caught up between "traditional life" and "modernity". This chapter appears to confirm the findings of an earlier study among the rural and urban Zaramo of Dar–es-Salaam, Tanzania (Swantz, 1979).

J. K. Githae's contribution in *Chapter 5* is partly polemical but represents an empirical case of the practice of traditional medicine. This chapter is included in this collection to demonstrate the patronage of traditional medicine and to show a possible framework for innovative adaptation within traditional medicine. Kikuyu traditional medicine appears to be going this direction (see also Chapter 11).

Chapter 6 by I. Sindiga discusses Luo therapy-seeking behaviour. Using case histories, in-depth interviews and observations of patients found consulting traditional healers, he sought to establish why patients go to traditional healers, to obtain profiles of patients seeking therapy in traditional medicine, to establish how choices of therapy are made and who makes such choice decisions, and to establish the pattern of consultation of the various medical systems. Sindiga found that the Luo seek therapy freely between the available medical systems and he explains that this behaviour, in the face of well articulated disease aetiologies, is partly a result of the confusion caused by the diffuse nature of disease symptoms. The difficulty in interpreting symptoms and determining the cause of a given episode of illness (whether naturalistic, supernatural or human-induced) will make people oscillate between traditional and modern medicine in order to maximize the chances of recovery.

E. A. Kawango also deals with traditional medicine among the Luo in *Chapter 7*. Utilizing field data from Siaya District, she discusses Luo remedies and therapies in maternal and child health.

The four chapters that follow cover traditional medicine among the Maasai, Abagusii, Abaluyia and Kikuyu. These case studies add depth and improve on the breadth of the subject covered in the book. In addition, they reveal that each community has multiple disease aetiologies thereby dispelling the myth of the supernatural as the only cause of disease in Africa. Also, disease, illness and misfortune are closely linked. Further, these case studies show that African traditional medicine has wide specializations with skilled medical experts. In general, the various case studies allow for cross-cultural comparisons of traditional medicine. In *Chapter 8*, Sindiga examines the place of traditional medicine in Maasai society. His overview of the subject probes the concept of disease causation and Maasai medical experts. He provides original data on the subject collected among the Kenya Maasai in Narok District. In *Chapter 9*, Sindiga also presents a case study of Gusii traditional medicine. This Chapter shows that the Abagusii have skilful surgeons who have performed delicate head trephining for centuries. The Gusii concept on what causes disease, illness and misfortune, and how this influences therapy-seeking behaviour, are also discussed.

Chapter 10 deals with the case of Luyia traditional medical practices whereby S. Wandibba focuses on Luyia disease aetiologies and the impact of colonialism on these. He discusses the contemporary status of traditional medicine in the Luyia community. An interesting issue which Wandibba brings out is the emergence of individuals who use the Bible in the divination process and then administer herbal remedies, perhaps a sign of the "modernization" of the Luyia traditional medicine.

Chapter 11 by Aseka, Kiriga, Sindiga and Kanunah, discusses the Kikuyu concept of disease and illness and the contemporary status of traditional medicine in that community. The authors observe that to become a Kikuyu medicinemen *(mũndũ mũgo)* requires painstaking training which culminates in formal initiation. The traditional medical practitioners must meet the highest vocational and ethical standards. However, contemporary Kikuyuland has undergone profound socio-economic changes emanating from contact with the West. As a result, traditional medical practice appears to be somewhat subdued in the rural areas. Nevertheless a modified form of Kikuyu medicine, based on herbal treatment, is becoming firmly established in Nairobi and other towns within Kikuyuland.

The three essays that follow by Baquar, Obado and Odera, and Kofi-Tsekpo deal with medicinal plants and drugs. In *Chapter 12,* S. R. Baquar calls for a systematic survey, collection, identification and documentation of medicinal herbs with a view of building a germplasm collection in the country, a view that is supported by Kofi-Tsekpo. He argues that Kenya is losing a lot of foreign exchange in importing drugs when its own environment is rich in herbal medicines. Baquar's general account of the history of the use of herbal medicines includes a discussion of herbal drugs that are universally used and their applications.

E. A. O. Obado and J. E. Odera discuss, in *Chapter 13*, the various methods of harvesting medicinal herbs in Nyanza and consider the effects on resource sustainability. The Luo have no local beliefs which favour the conservation of medicinal plants. Harvesting methods include extraction of whole plants and ring barking. The authors recommend the establishment of guidelines and rules for harvesting and conserving medicinal herbs. In addition, they call for comprehensive research and development agenda to foster the development of a pragmatic regime for crop renewal, harvesting and protocols for the sustainable management of medicinal plant germplasm.

W. M. Kofi-Tsekpo discusses the work going on at KEMRI in *Chapter 14*. This work should provide a rational scientific basis for formal accreditation to traditional medicines. KEMRI has been collaborating with traditional healers in the area of traditional drugs as a result of which herbal medicines have been tested and found to be effective for asthma, malaria, mild hypertension, diabetes, epilepsy, gout and arthritis. This is certainly an area where KEMRI should demonstrate strong leadership so that traditional medicines can be availed to the wider public. However, traditional healers are not always forthcoming with their drugs due to lack of legal protection. Another outstanding problem is that no mechanism exists for the evaluation and registration of traditional medicines. Such registration would require that the identity, safety and efficacy of the drugs be established.

In the final chapter (*Chapter 15*) Sindiga, Kanunah, Nyaigotti–Chacha and Mwangola, take a retrospective and prospective overview of traditional medicine in Africa. They identify three areas in which future work must be done in order to foster the development of traditional medicine. Attention must be directed to official health policy with regard to traditional medicine, professionalization of traditional medicine and creation of a *materia medica* in traditional medicine. The authors argue that legal recognition of traditional medicine, together with the issues of registration and licensing, are at the core of future development of traditional medicine in Africa.

A final thought

These essays represent the first Kenyan national effort to sensitize policy makers and the wider academy about the potentials and limitations of traditional medicine. As can be gleaned from the pages of this book, traditional medicine has been retarded since the colonial period. A lot of work requires to be done to salvage and give respectability to a health resource used by the majority of the African peoples. This is the imperative of traditional medicine.

REFERENCES

Akerele, O. 1987. "The Best of Both Worlds: Bringing Traditional Medicine Up to Date" *Social Science and Medicine* 24 No. 2: 177–181.

Ampofo, O. and F. D. Johnson-Romauld. 1987. "Traditional Medicine and Its Role in the Development of Health Services in Africa". Background paper for the technical discussions of the 25th, 26th and the 27th sessions of the Regional Committee for Africa. Brazzaville: World Health Organization.

Bennett, F. J. and J. Maneno (eds). 1986. *National Guidelines for the Implementation of Primary Health Care in Kenya.* Nairobi: Ministry of Health, the Non-Governmental Health Organizations of Kenya, WHO and UNICEF.

Caldwell, J.C. 1991. "The Soft Underbelly of Development: Demographic Transition in Conditions of Limited Economic Change". In *Proceedings of World Bank Annual Conference on Development Economics, 1990* edited by S. Fisher, D. De Tray and S. Shah. Washington D.C.: World Bank, pp. 207-253.

Oduory, T. M. 1991. "Preface", In *National Curriculum for Traditional Birth Attendants.* Nairobi: Division of Nursing and Division of Family Health in Conjunction with WHO and the Government of Belgium.

Erickson, R. J. et. al. 1989. "Medical Geography". In *Geography in America* edited by G. L. Gaile and C. J. Willmott. Columbus, Ohio: Merrill, pp. 425-450.

Feachem. R. G. and D. T. Jamison (eds). 1991. *Diseases and Mortality in Sub-Saharan Africa.* New York: Oxford.

Feachem, R. G., D. T. Jamison and E. R. Bos. 1991. "Changing Patterns of Disease and Mortality in Sub-Saharan Africa". In *Disease and Mortality in Sub–Saharan Africa* edited by R. G. Feachem and D. T. Jamison. New York: Oxford. pp. 3-27.

Golladay, F. and B. Liese, 1980. *Health Problems and Policies in Developing Countries.* World Bank Staff Working Paper No. 412. Washington D. C: World Bank.

Good, C. M. 1980. "A Comparison of Rural and Urban Ethnomedicine Among the Kamba of Kenya". In *Traditional Health Care Delivery in Contemporary Africa* edited by P. R. Ulin and M.H. Segall. Syracuse: Syracuse University. pp. 13-56.

________. 1987. *Ethnomedical Systems in Africa: Patterns of Traditional Medicine in Rural and Urban Kenya.* New York: Guilford Press.

Good, C. M. and V. N. Kimani. 1985. "Urban Traditional Medicine: A Nairobi Case Study". *East African Medical Journal* 57 No. 5:301-316.

Graham, W. J. 1991. "Maternal Mortality: Levels, Trends and Data Deficiencies". In *Disease and Mortality in Sub-Saharan Africa* edited by R. G. Feachem and D. T. Jamison. New York: Oxford. pp. 101-116.

Guo–Bin, L. 1987. "Traditional Medicine in the Western Pacific Region". *Report of the Second Meeting of Directors of WHO Collaborating Centres for Traditional Medicine, Beijing, China 16-20 November*. Geneva: WHO. pp 30-43.

Katz, S. H. and V. N. Kimani. 1982. "Why Patients go to the Traditional Healers." *East African Medical Journal* 59 No. 3: 170-174.

Kenya, Republic of. 1979. *Development Plan 1979–1983.* Nairobi: Government Printer.

________. 1980. *Turkana District Development Plan 1979-1983.* Nairobi: Ministry of Finance and Planning.

________. 1982. *The Integrated Rural Surveys 1976-79: Basic Report.* Nairobi: Central Bureau of Statistics.

________. 1984. *South Nyanza District Development Plan 1984-1988.* Nairobi: Ministry of Finance and Planning.

________. 1989. *Development Plan 1989-1993.* Nairobi: Government Government Printer.

_________. 1994 *National Development Plan for the Period 1994 to 1996.* Nairobi: Government Printer.

Kokwaro, J. O. 1976. *Medicinal Plants of East Africa.* Nairobi: East African Literature Bureau.

Mayer, J. D. 1982. "Medical Geography: Some Unresolved Problems". *Professional Geographer* 34 No. 3: 261-269.

McIvor, C. 1989. "Traditional Medicine in Zimbabwe". *The Courier* 115 (May-June): 19-20.

Nakajima, H. 1987. "Inaugural Address". *Report of the Second Meeting of Directors of WHO Collaborating Centre for Traditional Medicine, Beijing, China 16-20 November*. Geneva: WHO. pp. 5-7.

Nchinda, T. C. 1976. "Traditional and Western Medicine in Africa: Collaboration or Confrontation?" *Tropical Doctor* 6:133-135.

Ofosu-Amaah, S. 1991. "Disease in Sub-Saharan Africa: An Overview" In *Disease and Mortality in Sub-Saharan Africa* edited by R. G. Feachem and D. T. Jamison. New York: Oxford. pp. 119-121.

Phillips, D. R. 1985. "Directions for Medical Geography in the 1980s: Some Observations From the United Kingdom." *Social Science and Medicine* 20 No. 4: 404-407.

Pillsbury, B. L. K. 1979. *Reaching the Rural Poor: Indigenous Health Practitioners Are There Already*. AID Programme Evaluation Discussion Paper No. 1. Washington D.C.: USAID.

_________. 1982. "Policy and Evaluation Perspectives on Traditional Health Care Practitioners in National Health Care Systems". *Social Science and Medicine* 16 :1825-1834.

Preble, E. A. 1990. "Impact of HIV/AIDS on African Children." *Social Science and Medicine* 31 No. 6:671-680.

Swantz, M. L. 1979. "Community and Healing Among the Zaramo in Tanzania." *Social Science and Medicine* 13B:169-173.

Thairu, K. 1975. *The African Civilization*. Nairobi: East African Literature Bureau.

Twumasi, P. A. 1984. *Professionalisation of Traditional Medicine in Zambia*. Nairobi: IDRC.

Warren, D. M. 1988. "Utilizing Indigenous Healers in National Health Delivery Systems: The Ghananian Experiment". In *Making Our Research Useful: Case Studies in the Utilization of*

Anthropological Knowledge edited by J. van Willingen, B. Ryko-Bauer and A. MacElroy. Boulder: Westview.

World Bank. 1980. *Health Sector Policy Paper*. Washington D.C: World Bank.

_________. 1989. *Sub-Saharan Africa From Crisis to Sustainable Growth: A Long-Term Perspective Study*. Washington D.C: World Bank.

WHO. 1987. *The Promotion and Development of Traditional Medicine: Report of a WHO Meeting No. 622*. Geneva: WHO.

_________. 1985. *Report of the Consultation Approaches for Policy Development for Traditional Health Practitioners, Including Traditional Birth Attendants*. Geneva: WHO.

Chapter 2

AFRICAN ETHNOMEDICINE AND OTHER MEDICAL SYSTEMS

Isaac Sindiga

Introduction

This chapter discusses the conceptual foundations of African ethnomedicine and its relationship with other medical systems. This medical pluralism is the basis for inquiries into therapy–seeking and therapy-selecting behaviour of consumers of health services. Thus, the place of African ethnomedical systems can accurately be assessed.

Until about the 1970s, most studies concerned with traditional medicine in Africa linked it with beliefs, religion and ritual (Yoder, 1982). Such studies, pioneered by Evans-Pritchard (1937), uncritically observed that African disease aetiologies were basically moral and social (Yoder, 1982) – this scholarship followed the structural functionalist school of British anthropology.

Mutungi (1977) appears to have unwittingly followed British anthropology by focusing primarily on the role of the supernatural in disease causation*. According to him, the problem with witchcraft in traditional African societies "lies in the inseparability of such concepts as medicine; religion (faith); science and the phenomenon of witchcraft itself. These tend to form a unit which is difficult to grasp . . ."

Mutungi conceives too narrowly of witchcraft and fails to face the theoretical aspects of African disease, illness and misfortune aetiologies of which witchcraft is only a part (see Chapter 6). He does not examine the basis of African medical systems and borrows the Western lable of "witchdoctors" to refer to African traditional healers and writes in the following words:

---

* Onesmus K. Mutungi is a Kenyan law lecturer and a former Deputy Vice-Chancellor at the University of Nairobi.

> Witchdoctors (*awe* in Kamba) devote their activities to the care and healing of the sick by use of native herbs and the paraphernalia that go with such practices in the given society (Mutungi, 1977:xvi).

Part of the misunderstanding regarding the role of the African traditional healers emanates from the colonial times which is responsible for the negative approach to African traditional medicine. This includes the view that all healers are witch hunters practising "black magic" (Thairu, 1975).

Witchcraft refers to all the aspects of the use of mystical power to harm others in society (Mbiti, 1969) in which sense, witchcraft, sorcery, evil magic, evil eye, or whatever terminology it may be given, is evil. However, there is also "good magic" which represents the manipulation of mystical power by a traditional healer in the treatment process for the good of society (Mbiti, 1969:198). In this way, traditional healers serve to neutralize the power of sorcerers or witches which is harmful. This is only one facet of the work of traditional healers. Africans have diverse disease aetiologies which include "diseases of the air" or natural diseases and not just the supernatural. Another source of the misunderstanding may be attributed to lack of theoretical formulations of medical systems to allow an understanding of how each system is designed and conceptualized.

Medical Systems

Irwin Press (1980) has defined a medical system as a "patterned interrelated body of values and deliberate practices, governed by a single paradigm of the meaning, identification, prevention and treatment of sickness". A medical system must thus be conceived and designed in a particular way. In the words of Charles Leslie (1978: xii),

> Medical systems are social and cultural. In contrast to health systems, their boundaries are not those of biological populations, species and ecological networks; but of political organization and cultural exchange.

Each medical system has a number of attributes. These include; concept of disease causation, nosology, prophylaxis, therapy-seeking and therapy-selecting behaviour, therapy management and choice, range of practitioners (i.e. medical resources), practitioner specializations, travel for patients to see the practitioners and vice versa, diagnosis of health problem and therapy procedures and drugs and other pharmacopoeia (Yoder, 1982). These and other attributes of all medical systems make it possible to compare one system with another (Yoder, 1982:8). It also enables the simultaneous study of various systems. However, each medical system reflects part of the cultural and social patterning of the society of which it is part (Fabrega, 1975; 1982; Yoder, 1982). Yoder's (1982) warning that several criteria must be used when comparing various medical systems is certainly essential.

Ethnomedicine

Fabrega (1975:969) defines ethnomedicine as the study of the different ways in which people of various cultures perceive and cope with illness, including making a diagnosis and obtaining therapy. *Illness* refers to "a disvalued change in the adaptation functioning of an individual that gives rise to a need for corrective action" (Fabrega, 1982:239). This social definition of sickness, different from the malfunctioning of an organ (or *disease*), recognizes that *health* is adaptability (Meade, 1977:382) both of the individual and of the social group.

The ethnomedical approach to health problems is based on the notion that each cultural group handles its medical problems in a particular way "has its own world–view, traditions, values and institutions which have developed over time to handle disease and illness" (Last, 1986; Pillsbury, 1979; Fabrega, 1975; 1982; Good et al., 1979). Also, each culture has its own disease aetiologies, medical terminologies and classification, medical practitioners, and a whole range of pharmacopoeia. A people's beliefs and response to disease and illness are, therefore, not static but change with time (Good et. al., 1979:142).

The aggregate of a group's "beliefs, strategies, behaviour and interactions with ... environment that pertain to sickness, its management, and health status" may be referred to as that group's *ethnomedical system* (Good, 1987a: 17). An ethnomedical system then comprises "all the resources and responses available to a community in addressing its health problems, organized spatially and changing over time" (Good, 1987a:17). Thus, certain forms of Western medicine may be adopted or adapted into a group's ethnomedical system (Good, 1987b:237). However, the core concepts, beliefs and practices of the group remain.

The definitions of medical system and ethnomedical system show that the terms are synonymous although ethnomedicine tends to have the burden of appearing ethnocentric (Yoder, 1982:10). Nonetheless, the focus on ethnomedicine aims to arrive at an understanding of how a group or society's system of medicine functions, to delineate different types of systems of medicine, and ultimately to derive theories that explain how different systems of medicine operate and change (Fabrega, 1982:240-241).

Certain confusion is created by the use of the term *modern medicine* in reference to "Western medicine" or "biomedicine". Although this book assumes this usage, this does not purport that the so-called traditional medicine is not modern — in fact, "all medicine is modern . . . despite the setting in time, place and culture" (WHO, 1978:6). The assumption of the term "modern" for biomedicine as is the case (in this book) is predicated on the view that biomedicine quickly adopts innovations in the scientific and technological world (WHO, 1978:9). This is an advantage which traditional medicine perhaps enjoys only in a diminished way. It must be emphasized, however, that traditional medicine is part of culture which itself is always getting modified with time.

The solidifying of ethnomedical investigations is a result of the utilization of a new set of methodologies called *ethnoscience*. This approach, which was developed in the United States, allows social scientists to "accurately record indigenous knowledge and decision-making systems" (Warren and Green, 1988:6). Ethnoscientific studies were initially conducted in agricultural decision-making among various cultural groups (Knight, 1974; Newman, 1970; Nietschmann, 1973). The renewed interest in indigenous knowledge has led to the establishment of a Centre for Indigenous Knowledge for Agriculture and Rural Development (CIKARD) at the Iowa State University which has stimulated research into indigenous knowledge systems with a view to learning how cultural groups adapt to various facets of their environments. CIKARD is rapidly becoming a repository and reference centre for materials and ongoing activities in this field. In Europe, the Leiden Ethnosystems and Development Programme (LEAD) in the Netherlands has gained prominence in fostering indigenous knowledge and is supported in this task by the Centre for International Research and Advisory Networks (CIRAN) which also publishes the international journal, *Indigenous Knowledge and Development Monitor*.

African Ethnomedical Systems

As already noted, African ethnomedical systems define disease and illness within given social contexts. To begin with, traditional African medicine may be defined as the

> totality of all knowledge and practices, whether explicable or not, used in diagnosing, preventing or eliminating a physical, mental or social disequilibrium and which rely exclusively on past experience and observation handed down from generation to generation, verbally or in writing (Ampofo and Johnson–Romauld, 1978:38-39).

Thus, disease and illness are intricately interwoven in the social status of the group concerned. Fabrega (1975:972) describes the ethnomedical approach to health problems more explicitly: when a person contracts an illness or is attacked by a disease, he or she cannot perform his or her duties or functions within the social group. The group, comprising family members, neighbours and/or friends, is affected by the individual's illness and helps to select therapy for the patient. Among the Maasai, for example, a patient is first given traditional medicine at home (As part of education, every Maasai youth has to learn about the various diseases in the environment and grasp herbal drugs used for their treatment). When a patient fails to respond to home treatment, elders consult one another on therapy and recommend a specialized healer (See chapter 8).

Understanding the social significance of disease and illness is the key to comprehending ethnomedical systems. This view defines health as a state of "social wholeness" (Wisner, 1976:82). In the African context,

> disease is not merely something resulting from malfunctioning in this or that organ or a lesion therein . . . but essentially of a rupture of life's harmony, to be imputed either to a material cause instinct with some "intangible force" or directly to that intangible force itself. It is . . . necessary in traditional medical practice to confront the symptomatology and aetiology of diseases not only in the material but also in the immaterial world (Ampofo and Johnson-Romauld, 1978:40).

Indeed, medical practice "even within the most scientific contexts, continues to be largely a social art rather than a rigorous science" (Mechanic, 1968:19-20).

In ethnomedical systems, disease and misfortune are regarded as having socio-religious foundations. Consequently, the treatment process must go beyond addressing the symptomatology of disease to discovering its deep-seated causes and subsequent ways of preventing it from recurring (Mbiti, 1969:169-170). Although the classification is somewhat simplistic, the causes of disease and illness may be either natural (i.e. God-given) or unnatural (i.e. human induced) (IDRC, 1980; Mbiti, 1969). *Natural diseases* such as diarrhoea and skin rash in children, or rheumatism in older people (IDRC, 1980), may be treated either by modern medicine or by traditional medicine or by both. *Human-induced illness* on the other hand may be a result of sorcery, witchcraft, spirit disturbances or breaching socio-religious obligations and taboos especially with regard to the ancestors (living dead) (Whisson, 1974: 286; IDRC, 1980:12; Mbiti, 1969) and such disease must be referred to traditional healers. But disease and illness have multiple causes so that sometimes the symptoms are confusing thereby leading to pragmatic therapy-seeking, both in modern and in traditional medicine. This is demonstrated by the Luo case as shown in Chapter 6.

Diseases attributed to both naturalistic and supernatural causes can be treated by traditional healers who exist in each African village (Mbiti, 1969:166). A traditional healer may be defined as

> a person who is recognized by the community in which he lives as competent to provide health care by using vegetable, animal and mineral substances and certain other methods based on the social, cultural and religious background as well as on the knowledge, attitudes, and beliefs that are prevalent in the community regarding physical, mental and social well-being and the causation of disease and disability (Ampofo and Johnson-Romauld, 1978:39).

This all-encompassing definition suggests that traditional healers are "the friends, pastors, psychiatrists and doctors of traditional African villages and communities" (Mbiti, 1969:171). The traditional medical practitioners "symbolize the hopes of society; hopes of good health, protection and security from evil forces, prosperity and good fortune, and ritual cleansing when harm or impurities have been contracted" (Mbiti, 1969:171). Therefore, the traditional healer must be a morally upright person able to inspire trust among the citizenry and charge affordable fees (Mbiti, 1969:167). Such a healer commands much respect in his community.

Traditional healers have various specializations; there are herbalists, diviners, seers, spiritualists, traditional surgeons and birth attendants among other categories (IDRC, 1980; Ampofo and Johnson-Romauld, 1978; Mbiti 1969). A person may have one or more specializations; their knowledge and skills are based on years of careful empirical observations (IDRC, 1980).

The greatest advantage of African traditional medicine is its holistic approach to medical problems and misfortunes whereby both organic and psychological attributes of disease or illness are considered together. Swantz's study of the Zaramo of Tanzania shows that they conceive of life from the view of wholeness (*uzima*) which suggests "living in peace with one's fellow being and in harmony within oneself, in body and spirit". For this reason, disorders of the physical body reflect social disharmony hence the necessity for utilizing traditional and modern medicine at the same time (Swantz, 1979:169-170).

The psychological component of illness is brought out succinctly in the following passage:

> There is . . . incontrovertible evidence that at least a quarter of all adult patients seeking medical attention at primary health care level – i.e. dispensaries, health centres, out-patient departments, general practitioners - suffer primarily from a psychiatric condition. Another quarter will be suffering from a combination of psychiatric condition and organic condition. In other words, nearly half of all the patients seen at primary health care level have a psychiatric component to their illness *(East African Medical Journal,* 1987: 713).

Ordinarily, biomedical personnel do not concern themselves with the deep-seated causes of physical symptoms to disease. This is an area for the traditional healer.

Biomedicine

Biomedicine is the knowledge, practices, organization and social roles of medicine in Western cultures (Fabrega, 1975:969). Unlike ethnomedicine, the biomedical paradigm views disease and illness as physical or mechanical disorders with little relationship with a person's social and religious experiences (Good, 1980:96; Fabrega, 1975:969; Fabrega, 1982:241). In other words disease and illness are seen as mere organic malfunctioning. According to Fabrega (1975; 1982), disease is abstracted as a biological condition without the several social and psychological elements involved. In this view, disorders to the physical body may be caused by diet, genes, enzymes, organs, climate and social problems among others (Fabrega, 1982:241).

The aetiology of disease in the biomedical system leads to treatment which is restricted to controlling and eliminating physical symptoms.* This means that both doctor and the African patients use different value systems and frames of reference leading to the disillusionment of the patient with the treatment process. Inevitably the healing process is retarded.

Biomedicine (or Western medicine) has many constraints that include:

- inaccessibility both in physical distance and cost;
- shortage of drugs and equipment;
- inability to treat and cure certain diseases;
- impersonal care, (i.e. distance between medical staff and patient); and
- patients' expectation of instant cure (IDRC, 1980).

Dissatisfaction with biomedicine has led people, even in developed countries, to seek alternative therapies. Christie and Sandberg (1989) note that between a quarter to one fifth of the people in the Scandinavian countries, particularly Norway, now utilize alternative medicine. They seek treatment in acupuncture, homeopathy and chiropractic. Most patients move between biomedicine and alternative therapies.

---

* This is not to say that biomedicine does not concern itself with psychological problems of patients. The situation is that psychiatry tends to be a separate branch from general medical practice especially at the health centre level where most patients receive treatment.

Medical Pluralism

Medical pluralism is the "existence in a single society of differently designed and conceived medical systems" (Janzen, 1978: xviii). Such systems exist together and may compete with one another (Fabrega, 1982: 241-242). The significance of medical pluralism is in the understanding of the provision of health care within a given society. This is especially so in the area of decision-making with regard to seeking and selecting therapy.

Africans frequently utilize both traditional and modern medicine simultaneously for the same episode of illness or at different times for different illnesses (Alexander, 1985). People go to biomedical facilities when they believe that an illness is naturalistic. This is particularly so for various children's diseases. On the other hand, people will turn to traditional healers when they conceive an illness to be caused by human-induced forces. Whatever the case, Africans are quite flexible in seeking treatment. Ampofo and Johnson-Romauld (1978:51) state it in the following way:

> The African peoples believe in traditional medicine and it is not uncommon to see patients in hospitals permitting themselves to be treated by modern medicine during the day and having recourse to the recipes of traditional medicine at night.

As argued in Chapter 6 in the case of the Luo, such behaviour is probably motivated by a desire to maximize chances of regaining health especially in view of conflicting symptoms of naturalistic and human-induced illness.

Although many African communities categorize disease and illness according to cause, they see traditional and modern medicine as complementary. Among the Luvale of Zambia, barrenness, postpartum weakness, madness and a number of other illnesses are reserved for traditional medicine (Spring, 1980). Similarly, the Keiyo and the Marakwet of Kenya see women infertility, infantile diarrhoea, trephining of fractured skulls and mental illness as best handled in traditional medicine, whereas obstetric cases, acute respiratory infections, trachoma, accidents and fevers belong to modern medicine (Nyamwaya, 1981; Kipkorir, 1980). This dichotomy, however, exists only at the belief level. When faced with an actual episode of illness a person may move from one traditional healer to another and from traditional medicine to health centre or hospital and vice versa (Nyamwaya, 1981).

Because of the existence of medical pluralism and because of patients' utilization of the different systems, separately or jointly, it is necessary to study the existing systems in order to see how they can be brought to work together for the enhancement of health within primary health care. It is true that the various medical systems may compete with one another (Fabrega, 1982:241-242); nevertheless, people see and utilize them in a complementary or even supplementary way.

Cooperation Between African Traditional Medicine and Modern Medicine

Are there possibilities of cooperation between African traditional medicine and modern medicine (biomedicine)?

When the WHO recommended the use of traditional medicine in national health care services, it strongly urged cooperation between ethnomedicine and biomedicine. At the introduction of the latter no effort was made for the two systems to work together; they tended to develop separately (Akerele, 1987) hence there is little communication between the practitioners of the two systems. In fact, African traditional medicine was suppressed and then ignored in the European colonies.

As a prerequisite to cooperation between the two systems, there should be detailed understanding of both systems and this should include their contributions to health care at all levels in various communities. And this is the approach taken in this book. To be of value to the peoples of developing countries, the various medical systems must overcome the problem of communication and reach certain accommodation with regard to the language and values held by the other.

It is clear that, whereas traditional healers recognize biomedicine and refer their patients to it, the reverse is not true. Therefore, there is need for training (i.e. reorienting) biomedical personnel to appreciate the potential of the other party whilst training traditional healers to enhance their abilities and recognize their own limitations.

Biomedical personnel complain of a myriad weaknesses with traditional medicine. Some of the alleged weakness are genuine whereas others are superfluous; traditional medicine is part of culture which is not static but changes with time and place. The real problem of acceptability of traditional medicine across the board in any one society is perhaps the great emphasis on Western medicine (Pillsbury, 1979:14). The colonial rejection of traditional medicine as magic, ritual and witchcraft meant that the modernization process had led to the destruction of certain cultural attributes among which is traditional medicine (see Chapters 10 and 11).

Today, there are two groups of people in any African society - those with formal Western education and those with indigenous informal education. In general, the younger people with Western education may have values which may be in conflict with those held by their less literate elders over the role of traditional medicine. In certain circumstances, the process of Westernization has gone hand in hand with Christianization. The latter discourages traditional medicine and has almost always wished to replace it with biomedicine.

Another impediment to integration is the perceived and actual competition for clients. For this reason, there has been little desire in the biomedical establishments (which control health ministries in various countries) to support research in traditional medicine.

Problems with traditional medicine

- It does not keep up with scientific and technological advancement.
- Its methods, techniques, medicines and even training are often kept secret.
- It is difficult to diagnose chronic illness in time.
- The rational use of traditional medicine is not well defined; it relies on mysticism and intangible forces, for example, witchcraft.
- Some aspects are based on spiritual and moral principles which are difficult to explicate
- It lacks "measured" doses of drugs; sometimes the side effects of a combination of herbal medicines used is not known.
- It has an alleged low quality of care because of lack of regulatory mechanisms including control and licensing.
- It keeps no written registers of patients hence difficult to evaluate. This is especially so for African systems.
- It experiences loss of knowledge or errors occasioned by large numbers of herbs and other pharmacopoeia; and diseases to be treated are many.

SOURCES: WHO, 1978; Ampofo and Johnson-Romauld, 1978; Kokwaro, 1976; Pillsbury, 1979; Nakajima, 1987; Mbiti, 1969.

Traditional Medicine, Therapy-seeking Behaviour and Medical Geography

As shown earlier, the increasing interest in traditional medicine owes to the inadequacy of the spatial coverage of modern medicine and hence the need to incorporate traditional medicine in national health care delivery systems. The major impediment to traditional medicine's participation in official health care, at least initially, is lack of data on various aspects of traditional medical practices (WHO, 1978:37). Research data required in several aspects of traditional medicine include;

- census of traditional healers in practice specifying their specializations,
- traditional medical systems, procedures, skills, technology and their philosophical underpinnings,
- medicinal substances used especially plants,
- diseases successfully treated in traditional medicine,
- organization of traditional medicine in local communities,
- utilization of traditional healers in health services,
- manpower needs, and
- metaphysics and parascientific areas such as cosmology, astrology, parapsychology, hypnosis, religious incantations, and meditation (WHO, 1978:33-37).

Despite the many potential areas of research in traditional medicine, there have been few geographic studies on ethnomedical systems in various communities (Mayer, 1982:267; Paul, 1985: 403). Geographers are particularly suited to conduct research on the utilization patterns of traditional medical systems (Phillips, 1985:406).

Investigating patient utilization patterns requires basic locational data for which geographers are trained (Good, 1977:70). Another contribution that geographers can make is to indicate the distribution of medical problems, perceived or real, both in local areas and at regional and national scales (Vogel, 1974). Their mapping technique is capable of showing distribution of diseases and other health problems, knowledge which could be used to make decisions on ameliorative action. The initial task would be to gather data on all the health resources available within a community. The subsequent painting showing medical landscapes of a given community will enable policy-makers to make meaningful plans for health service delivery (Good, 1977). Thereafter, having established the availability and accessibility of various medical systems within a community, people's utilization patterns of the services and the rationale for their usage plus their perceptions of the various systems, it will be possible to recommend ways through which traditional medical systems may be incorporated in national health care services.

REFERENCE

Akerele, O. 1987. "The Best of Both Worlds: Bringing Traditional Medicine up to date". *Social Science and Medicine* 24 No. 2:177-181.

Alexander, G. A. 1985. "A survey of Traditional Medical Practices used for the Treatment of Malignant Tumours in an East African Population" *Social Science and Medicine* 20 No. 7:54-59.

Ampofo, O. and J. D. Johnson-Romauld. 1987. "Traditional Medicine and Its Role in the Development of Health Services in Africa. "Background paper for the Technical Discussions of the 25th, 26th and 27th Sessions of the Regional Committee for Africa. Brazzaville: WHO.

Christie, V. M. and E. Sandberg. 1989. "A Dialogue Between Practitioners of Alternative (Traditional) Medicine and Modern (School) Medicine in Norway." Paper to the Eleventh International Conference on the Social Sciences and Medicine, Leeuwenhorst Congress Centre, the Netherlands, 24-28 July.

East African Medical Journal. 64 No. 11 (1987): 713-714.

Evans-Pritchard, E.E. 1937. *Witchcraft, Oracle and Magic Among the Azande.* Oxford: Oxford University Press.

Fabrega, H. 1975. "The Need for an Ethnomedical Science" *Science* 189 No. 4207: 969-975.

_________. 1982. "A Commentary on African Systems of Medicine". In *African Health and Healing Systems: Proceedings of a Symposium* edited by P. S. Yoder. Los Angeles: Crossroads Press. pp. 237-252.

Good, C. M. 1977. "Traditional Medicine: An Agenda for Medical Geography" *Social Science and Medicine* 11:705-713.

_________. 1980."Ethnomedical Systems in Africa and the LDCs: Key Issues for the Geographer". In *Conceptual and Methodological Issues in Medical Geography* edited by M.S. Meade. Chapel Hill: University of North Carolina. pp 93-116.

_________. 1987a."Community Health in Tropical Africa: Is Medical Pluralism a Hindrance or a Resource?" In *Health and Disease in Tropical Africa: Geographical and Medical Viewpoints* edited by R. Akhtar. London: Gordon and Breach. pp. 13-50.

_________. 1987b. *Ethnomedical Systems in Africa*. New York: Guilford.

Good, C. M. et al. 1979. "The Interface of Dual Systems of Health Care in the Developing World: Toward Policy Initiatives in Africa" *Social Science and Medicine* 13D:141-154.

IDRC. 1980. *Traditional Medicine in Zaire: Present and Potential Contribution to the Health Services.* (Ottawa: IDRC.

Janzen, J. M. 1978. *The Quest for Therapy: Medical Pluralism in Lower Zaire*. Berkeley: University of California.

Kipkorir, B. E. 1980. "African Traditional Medicine and Kalenjin Medicine and Surgery." *Hekima* 1:23-36.

Knight, C. G. 1974. *Ecology and Change: Rural Modernization in an African Community*. New York: Academic Press.

Kokwaro, J. O. 1976. *Medicinal Plants of East Africa*. Nairobi: East African Literature Bureau.

Last, M. 1986. "The Professionalisation of African Medicine: Ambiguities and Definitions". In *The Professionalisation of African Medicine* edited by M. Last and G. L. Chavunduka. Manchester: Manchester University Press. pp. 1-19.

Leslie, C. 1978. "Foreword" In *The Quest for Therapy: Medical Pluralism in Lower Zaire* edited by J. M. Janzen. Barkeley: University of California. pp. xi-xv

Mayer, J. D. 1982. "Medical Geography: Some Unresolved Problems" *Professional Geographer*, 34 No. 3:261-269.

Mbiti, J. S. 1969. *African Religions and Philosophy*. London: Heinemann.

Meade, M. S. 1977. "Medical Geography as Human Ecology: The Dimension of Population Movement" *Geographical Review* 67 No. 4: 379-393.

Mechanic, D. 1968. *Medical Sociology: A Selective View.* New York: Free Press.

Mutungi, O. K. 1977. *The Legal Aspects of Witchcraft in East Africa with Particular Reference to Kenya*. Nairobi: East African Literature Bureau.

Nakajima, H. 1987. "Inaugural Address". In *Report of the Second Meeting of Directors of WHO Collaborating Centre for Traditional Medicine, Beijing China 16-20 November.* Geneva: WHO. pp. 5-7.

Newman, J. L. 1970. *The Ecological Basis for Subsistence Change Among the Sandawe of Tanzania.* Washington D.C.: National Academy of Science.

Nietschmann, B. 1973. Between Land and Water: The Subsistence Ecology of the Miskito Indians, Eastern Nicaragua. New York: Seminar Press.

Nyamwaya, D. 1981. "Complementarity in Health Care: The Case of Elgeyo-Marakwet District". In *Kerio Valley: Past, Present and Future* edited by B.E. Kipkorir, R. C. Soper and J. W. Ssenyonga. Nairobi: University of Nairobi. pp. 120-131.

Paul, B. K. 1985. "Approaches to Medical Geography: An Historical Perspective" *Social Science and Medicine* 20 No. 4: 399-404.

Phillips, D. R. 1985. "Directions for Medical Geography in the 1980s: Some Observations From the United Kingdom". *Social Science and Medicine* 20 No. 4:404-407.

Press, I. 1980. "Problems in the Definition and Classification of Medical Systems". *Social Science and Medicine* 14B:45-57.

Spring, A. 1980. "Traditional and Biomedical Health Care Systems in Northwest Zambia: A Case of the Luvule". In *Traditional Health Care Delivery in Contemporary Africa* edited by P. R. Ulin and M. H. Segall. Syracuse: Syracuse University. pp. 57-79.

Swantz, M. L. 1979. "Community and Healing Among the Zaramo in Tanzania". *Social Science and Medicine* 13B:169-173.

Thairu, K. 1975. The African Civilization. Nairobi: East African Literature Bureau.

Vogel, L. C. 1974. "Epidemiology and Medical Geography". In *Health and Disease in Kenya* edited by L.C. Vogel et al. Nairobi: East African Literature Bureau. pp. 3-7.

Warren, D. M. and E. C. Green. 1988. "Linking Biomedical and Indigenous African Health Delivery Systems: An Assessment of Collaborative Efforts During the 1980s". Paper presented at the Conference on Ethnomedical Systems in Sub-Saharan Africa. 1-4 June. Leiden: Leiden University.

Whisson, M. C. 1974. "Some Aspects of Functional Disorders Among the Kenya Luo." In *Magic, Faith and Healing: Studies in Primitive Psychiatry Today* edited by A. Kiev. New York: Free Press. pp. 293-304.

Wisner, B. 1976. "Health and the Geography of Wholeness". In Contemporary Africa: *Geography and Change* edited by C. G. Knight and J. L. Newman. Englewood Cliffs: Prentice Hall. pp. 81-100.

WHO. 1978. The Promotion and Development of Traditional Medicine: Report of a WHO Meeting No. 622. Geneva: WHO.

Yoder, P. S. 1982. "Issues in the Study of Ethnomedical Systems in Africa". In African Health and Healing Systems: Proceedings of a Symposium edited by P. S. Yoder. Los Angeles: Crossroads Press. pp. 1-20.

Chapter 3

A CASE FOR TRADITIONAL MEDICINE IN OFFICIAL HEALTH SERVICES
Flogging a Dead Horse?

David O. Nyamwaya

Introduction

Soon after independence, and particularly during the 1970s, a lively debate raged in many African countries regarding the place of African traditional medicine in the development of health services. Those involved in the debate were mainly academicians joined by a few liberal policy-makers. The debate led to some research initiatives and the publication of a number of academic papers, for example, Janzen (1974), Harrison (1974), Chavunduka (1978) and Ademuwagun et. al. (1979). The purpose of these initiatives was to make the case for the recognition of traditional medicine as a critical component of national health systems. In Kenya, the case was made and indeed the government, in its 1979 National Development Plan, stated that:

> Traditional medicine and health care are an important part of the life of the people in the rural areas. However, more information is needed and will be collected during this plan period with regard to both its substantive aspect and its potential link with government institutions ... Further, considerations will be given to the manpower aspects of the traditional sector, for instance, the extent to which certain cadres of selected traditional sector practitioners such as midwives, might be encouraged to serve in Government health institutions in the rural areas (Kenya, 1979:136).

This tacit recognition was subsequently complemented with further articulation of what needed to be done to facilitate utilization of aspects of traditional medicine in official health service delivery. This was done through the guidelines on primary health which came out in 1986 and 1991 (Maneno and Mwanzia, 1991).

In the light of what has been observed in different parts of Kenya since 1979, it is justifiable to state that, in spite of the policy enunciations mentioned above, not much has been done in terms of full recognition for traditional medicine, provision of support for its technical development through research and development, and the development of registration and certification procedures for the practitioners. Therefore, the issue of placing traditional medicine in its rightful position in Kenya's official health care system is far from settled. While the matter awaits settlement, most Kenyans continue to use traditional medicine in a variety of ways.

In this chapter, a situational analysis of the diverse utilization of traditional medicine is done, the gaps calling for further action identified (these gaps include legal, technical and organizational aspects), problems arising from the gaps are defined and finally, a proposal for the recognition of, support to and regulation for traditional medicine is made. It should be pointed out that for purposes of the discussion, traditional medicine is assumed to include both lay-therapies and the services provided by indigenous medical practitioners. It should be stated further that discussion of harmful forms of traditional medicine (such as those practised by the so-called "witchdoctors") is not included. Granted that there are some practitioners who combined both useful therapeutic intervention and harmful practices, the focus is on the former aspect.

The Existence and Use of Traditional Medicine in Kenya

The exact proportion of the Kenyan population which uses traditional medicine is not clearly established, but as of 1991 it is estimated to be between zero and 75 per cent (Maneno and Mwanzia, 1991). Research carried out in over 10 districts indicates that traditional medicine is considered as an integral component of the health services available for use in the management of various medical conditions and the prevention of some of these conditions. Traditional perceptions of health and disease are widespread in Kenya, even among people who routinely use Western-type medicine (Nyamwaya, 1992).

Among all the communities studied, it is believed that, as a biological entity, the human body may malfunction due to old age, invasion by organisms such as worms, or due to injuries sustained from accidents. It is also believed that bad food, weather changes and poisonous substances can also affect the body and cause illness.

Illnesses that are seen to arise from normal biological processes in or affecting the human body are responded to in a matter-of-fact way. Herbal or other concoctions are administered as appropriate - orally, as ointments, or through incisions on the skin. Prevention of this kind of body malfunction is seen to lie in the administration of the appropriate medicines or physiotherapy. Still on the biological level, an illness may be thought to be caused by an individual's "too many thoughts, ideas or plans in the mind". This reference of a seemingly psychological nature may not be stretched to include interpersonal or spiritual forces.

Health and illness among the communities studied include both the "how" component (as discussed above) and a "why" component. The how component relates to the biological factors contributing to the causation of an illness and the interventions deemed appropriate to eradicate the illness. The why component refers to the people's explanation with regard to the particularity of an illness and which relates to social and spiritual factors that are seen to be relevant to the timing of an illness. Social factors include breach of taboo, effects of curse and dishonour to others. Spiritual factors include God's punishment for individual or communal sins or affliction by ancestral spirits.

Several types of indigenous health practitioners exist in Kenya, but there is much confusion regarding the definition and functions of the indigenous practitioners. Terms such as "witchdoctor", "shaman", "healer", "indigenous practitioner" and many others are used interchangeably to denote a wide variety of practitioners. First it should be noted that there is a distinction between practitioners whose role involves the treatment of illness, and those who are believed to use supernatural powers to cause illness. In this chapter, only those who help to eradicate or cope with illness are dealt with.

A second distinction with regard to indigenous practitioners is based on their different categories which though overlapping in some instances, cannot be subsumed under one term; only generic terms such as healer or practitioner can be used. In any society, there are several categories and types of health specialists– herbalists, surgical herbalists, physiotherapists, birth attendants and psychosocial specialists.

Many scholars, most notably Romanucci-Ross (1977), have implied that for every society which uses both indigenous and cosmopolitan forms of therapy, there is a "hierarchy of resort" indicating the normal sequencing in the use made of existing health service alternatives (see also Chapter 6). While it is possible to plot a hierarchy of resort for a given illness, research experience indicates that individuals and families respond to the occurrence of a given illness in ways that are unique to them, and this response is influenced by a number of factors whose relative importance varies over time and space. It is, therefore, not useful to attempt to define a hierarchy of resort chart for any given society. What is important is an understanding of the factors which influence the choice of a specific therapeutic alternative. The diverse ways in which indigenous and cosmopolitan medicine interact are discussed in the coming section.

Basic to the hierarchy of resort in respect of the interaction between cosmopolitan and indigenous medicine, is the assumption that most societies dichotomize illness. It is usually argued that people make a clear distinction between illnesses which can be treated by cosmopolitan medicine (by the *mzungu*, the white man) and those which can be treated by indigenous medicine. It is argued further that any illness belonging to the *mzungu* category is referred to the cosmopolitan health facilities, while an illness which belongs to the other category is referred to the indigenous practitioners. Studies in many Kenyan societies over a long period indicate that this dichotomy is mainly cognitive. At the behavioural level, any dichotomization is rarely maintained.

A close examination of health-seeking behaviour in Kenyan societies from the lay perspective reveals that indigenous and cosmopolitan medicine can interact in four main forms and an analysis of the interaction reveals how people use both types of medicine even for the same illness.

The first form of interaction can be described as *sequential zig-zag*. In this form of relationship, a patient may start using either of the two forms and move on to the other and then return to the form that he had used initially. Thus, there is oscillation between the two types of medicine as the illness develops. This process can continue for any period of time.

The second form of interaction between the two forms of medicine can be described as *supplementary* and this relationship exists in cases where only one of the two forms of medicine can be used for the management or prevention of a condition. For example, among the Kikuyu, Abagusii, Kamba, Pokot and Kuria, the uvula is excised as a way of treating chronic coughing and to speed up normal human growth. This kind of therapy is seen to belong only to indigenous medicine. On the other hand, X-rays are used in cosmopolitan medicine, but not in indigenous medicine. In these two examples, there is a supplementary relationship in that the intervention within one form of medicine is regarded as one that is extra in the other. Cosmopolitan health care providers do not use uvula excision for the purpose it is used for in indigenous medicine. Likewise, X-rays are not used in indigenous medicine.

A third form of interaction may be described as one of *competition*. For example, in cases of acute ailments which are believed to be of only a biological nature, an individual or family decides to pursue either form of therapy depending on the importance of various factors (these will be discussed later). An example is indigestion which can be treated with liver salt bought over the counter or with an indigenous herbal mixture. If the condition persists, the patient can consult a nurse at a nearby dispensary or a herbalist. The interaction can, however, shift to the first form described.

A fourth, and by far the most important, form of interaction is that of *complementarity,* whereby people consider both types of medicine as necessary for complete healing to occur. The complementary relationship is common when chronic illnesses that are thought to involve psychosocial and spiritual factors occur; for example, a patient may be admitted in a cosmopolitan hospital, a specific diagnosis made and proper treatment effected. If the patient or his family thinks that psychosocial or spiritual factors are involved, a therapeutic ceremony may be performed at home. Such a ceremony is considered important in the healing process. Another example of complementarity is that of preventive care. It is now generally understood that immunization is necessary for child health. Besides taking children for immunization, most mothers also take indigenous measures to protect the child from malevolent individuals and spirits, protection that involves the use of *materia medica* or the wearing of charms and amulets.

The above discussion indicates that traditional medicine is used not only widely, but also in very close conjunction with Western medicine. This position calls for a proper understanding of traditional therapies and practitioners to facilitate consumer satisfaction.

Outstanding Issues on Traditional Medicine in Kenya

The legal standing of traditional medicine in Kenya is not quite clear. On the one hand are the policy statements mentioned earlier in the chapter and on the other, is the lack of a specific statutory provision on traditional medicine.

Traditional medical practitioners in several parts of Kenya complain of harassment by administrative personnel because the latter claim that traditional medicine is illegal, a notion that stems from a misinterpretation of the Witchcraft Ordinance (1925) which has for a long time been assumed to regulate traditional medical practice. However, most legal experts argue that the Ordinance does not really relate to beneficial therapeutic practice. It reads:

> Any person who holds himself out as a witchdoctor able to cause fear, annoyance or injury to another in mind, person or property, or who pretends to exercise any kind of supernatural power, witchcraft, sorcery or enchantment calculated to cause such fear, annoyance or injury shall be guilty of an offence and shall be liable to imprisonment of either description for a term not exceeding five years.

Due to this unclear legal status, many prominent people make use of the traditional medical care discretely fearing the social and legal sanctions which could result from public exposure.

Technically, traditional medicine lacks the scientific research support essential to any line of specialization; there is no comprehensive programme of research into traditional medical concepts, therapeutic strategies and pharmacopoeia. True, there are some individual researchers engaged in research into traditional medicine, but there is little coordination of these efforts. Due to lack of technical support to traditional medical practitioners, many harmful practices and toxic substances are used widely but the users and the practitioners are unaware of the dangers. Such harmful practices and substances should be identified and discouraged.

Lack of proper technical support for traditional medicine prevents further development/refinement of therapeutic procedures and substances. This is a serious ethical dilemma; if there be traditional medical procedures and substances which can be used in the management of medical conditions, such should be promoted for use by the general population. Failure to promote such procedures/substances goes against medical ethics.

Traditional practitioners need support in terms of training in basic disease prevention and management skills as well as general technology. Such support could be offered through in-service training or pre-service courses. At the moment, only herbalists and traditional birth attendants (TBAs) receive some training in aspects of primary health care (PHC). Lack of appropriate training, thus implies below optimal functioning by traditional practitioners.

It is important for traditional medical practitioners to operate within a clearly defined organizational framework. This framework is lacking in Kenya. There is no government-related structural arrangement to facilitate regulation of traditional medicine. There are no clear guidelines for certification and registration. There is an association of traditional healers, but the association tends to cater only for those practitioners with a propensity for publicity, mainly as a way of attracting clients; publicity-shy practitioners have not joined the association, which is itself an expensive undertaking costing upward of KShs. 1,000 per practitioner.

Lack of organizational structures and procedures makes it difficult to control malpractice among the practitioners which is reported frequently. For example, clients are lured into paying colossal sums of money for "cures" relating to incurable conditions such as cancer and AIDS. This lack of professional regulations on practice therefore leads to overcharging. Besides, there are not any generally accepted rates for the management of the same conditions by different practitioners and such a situation facilitates the thriving of quacks in traditional medicine.

Negative Effects of Unrecognized, Unregulated Traditional Medicine

The existence of traditional medicine that is not fully recognized and that receives little technical support, with hardly any effective regulations, has many negative effects. Delayed referral of cases requiring complicated surgical intervention tends to occur from time to time, because some traditional practitioners claim to treat all medical conditions. Such claims give the patient a false sense of hope.

A number of the drugs used by traditional practitioners have adverse effects. Moreover, the damage done to patients' health by such drugs is not even known. These drugs need to be studied so that those which are harmful are discouraged.

Due to lack of recognition and regulation of traditional medicine, there is now a proliferation of poorly trained practitioners who are not controlled by either the traditional social system or the modern government administration. Clandestine services can be abused easily because there is no system of sanctions affecting the activities. Users of such services do not necessarily distinguish between legitimate and clandestine forms of services.

The above situations reinforce the negative attitudes of administrators and Western-type health workers towards the traditional practitioners. In order to facilitate effective use of traditional medicine within the context of official Western health care, it is important that a number of policy, technical and organizational arrangements be effected.

Improving Traditional Medicine as a Component of Official Health Care

In present day Kenya, traditional medicine flourishes unrecognized, unsupported and unregulated by the government or any other institution and the resulting problems have been highlighted above. This is a proposition that, in order for traditional medicine to have an even bigger impact on the health of Kenyans than it is doing now, it should have full official recognition by the government and receive appropriate technical and other support, and that mechanisms for regulating this form of health care be developed. A call for such attention to traditional medicine by the government is necessary because the government sets and controls all policy relating to health development in the country. Recognition, support and regulation can provide additional legitimacy for traditional medicine, a condition for its further development and use by the public.

Before proposing some changes needed to facilitate the utilization of traditional medicine in official health care, there is need to discuss the question as to whether this refers to cooperation or incorporation of this form of health care with its Western counterpart. Cooperation between traditional practitioners and Western-type medical practitioners is something that is quite possible in the Kenyan context. In this situation, neither party is required to change its approaches to disease management or even the basic concepts of health and illness. Success or failure of cooperation between traditional and Western-type of practitioners depends very much on the individuals concerned and the institution in which they work. It is proposed that such cooperation be fostered to:

- facilitate exchange of information on diagnosis and use of drugs for the management of illness;
- enable the traditional practitioners acquire an understanding of basic ideas about primary health care and their role in it;
- enable Western-type practitioners acquire knowledge about the kind of treatment their patients may undergo before seeking cosmopolitan health care; and,
- improve the psychosocial aspects of therapy through referral of patients from traditional to cosmopolitan practitioners.

Some scholars think that traditional medicine, or at least aspects of it, should be incorporated into the existing official health care system (Ademuwagun, 1979:158). In my view, incorporation of traditional medicine into the existing official health care system raises a number of issues:

- Western-type of practitioners control resources within the Ministry of health - it is unlikely that they would be willing to share the resources which they already consider to be too limited.
- The two types of medicine are based on quite different concepts of health and illness which may conflict in some cases.
- Management of patients using both types of medicine and in the same place is likely to cause problems.
- Most western-type of practitioners look down upon their traditional counterparts - it may, therefore, be difficult for the two parties to operate on an equal footing.
- Western medicine emphasizes formal school-type education while traditional medicine emphasizes apprenticeship. In a situation of incorporation, it may be difficult to agree on training requirements.

It is proposed that a specific statute be enacted to facilitate the operation of traditional medicine in Kenya and should cover issues such as:

- financing of traditional medicine,

- registration and certification,
- training of practitioners,
- quality control,
- research and development, and
- interaction with Western-type of medicine.

It is proposed further that the government and relevant non-governmental organizations (NGOs) set aside resources and develop a mechanism for facilitating technical development of traditional medicine. Such development should include:

- chemical analysis of drugs and study of their pharmacology,
- documentation of the therapeutic techniques used by traditional practitioners with a view to promoting those which have proved to be efficacious, and
- development of training curricula.

It is important for the government to develop mechanisms and structures for regulating traditional medicine the same way it is done for Western-type medicine. This regulatory mechanisms and structures should include:

- rules of training, certification and registration,
- professional ethical standards,
- professional bodies,
- organizational structure - defining hierarchical and horizontal relationships, and
- fee for service structure.

The traditional practitioners should participate very actively in the development of the above regulatory mechanisms and structures.

Conclusion

While research and other evidence indicate that traditional medicine is widely used in Kenya, its use is largely informal and occurs outside the official health care system. This form of health care interacts closely with Western-type health care.

Although there is no direct interference with traditional medicine in the legal and administrative senses, number of issues are yet to be sorted out to enable the speciality to develop and benefit the people of Kenya more. It is proposed that action be taken by the government and relevant NGOs to help put traditional medicine in its right place in Kenya's health development. The required action needs to be catalyzed by the work of researchers who should delineate the issues involved. The horse is therefore not dead – the matter needs even more serious attention now than before because of the escalating costs of Western-type medicine.

REFERENCES

Ademuwagun, Z.A. et al. (eds). 1979. *African Therapeutic Systems*. Waltham, Massachusetts: Cross Roads Press.

Ademuwagun, Z. A. 1979. "Problems and Prospect of Legitimizing and Integrating Aspects of Traditional Health Care Systems and Methods With Modern Medical Therapy: The Igbo-ora Experience". In *African Therapeutic Systems* edited by Z.A. Ademuwagun et al. Waltham, Massachusetts: Cross Roads Press. pp. 158-164.

Chavunduka, G. L. 1978. *Traditional Healers and the Shona Patient*. Salisbury: Mambo Press.

Bennett, F. J. and J. Maneno. 1986. *National Guidelines for the Implementation of Primary Health Care in Kenya*. Nairobi: Ministry of Health WHO and UNICEF.

Kenya, Government of. 1925. *The Witchcraft Ordinance, Cap 67, Laws of Kenya* (revised 1962 and 1981). Nairobi: Government Printer.

Kenya, Government of. 1979. *Development Plan 1979-1983*. Nairobi: Government Printer.

Harrison, I. E. 1974. "Traditional Healers: A Neglected Source of Health Manpower" *Rural Africana* 26: 5-16.

Janzen, J. M. 1974. "Pluralistic Legitimisation of Therapy Systems in Contemporary Zaire." *Rural Africana* 26:105-122.

Maneno, J. and J. Mwanzia 1991. *12 Years of Primary Health Care in Kenya.* Nairobi: Ministry of Health, WHO and UNICEF.

Nyamwaya, D. 1992. *African Indigenous Medicine: An Anthropological Perspective for Policy Makers and Primary Health Care Managers.* Nairobi: African Medical and Research Foundation.

Romanucci-Ross, L. 1977. "The Hierarchy of Resort in Curative Practices: The Admiralty Islands, Melanesia." In *Culture, Disease and Healing: Studies in Medical Anthropology* edited by D. Landy et al. New York and London: Macmillan Publishing Co.

Chapter 4

CONFIDENCE IN TRADITIONAL HEALERS

Richard M. Swiderski

The person who is ill is taken to a witchdoctor. The witchdoctor starts talking about somebody bewitching the sick man. He states that the person responsible for his illness is his neighbour. The witchdoctor plucks out what seems to be snake ribs from the ill man's head. Under instructions, the family of the ill man unearths several bones, some teeth and hair from their doorstep. The witchdoctor says all these are works of the neighbour, who is said to have been behind the sickness of the man. One white bull, a white sheep and two white cocks are offered as a fee to the witchdoctor. Instructions are given that food should be offered to their ancestors two days on full moons. Some herbs are part of the medication. Witchdoctors are the ones who act as mediators between the people, their ancestors and gods. This is when trouble or when members of the society have abused their privileges or wronged their ancestors. It is witchdoctors who alert the people on coming disasters, interpreting them as part of punishments. They are the ones to offer alternatives and carry them out like sacrifices and offerings.

This passage is by a young Kamba man describing the role of one type of traditional healer in his society. He refers to the healer by the English word "witchdoctor" which has a specific meaning in contemporary Kenyan English, of someone capable of witchcraft, but using that skill or power to heal. The nature of the illness, the identity of the afflicted person, and even the specific performance of the treatment are secondary to the broad social context of the witchdoctor's activity. He works to rectify relations within a small local community: the illness is not a disease (Kleinman, 1978: 661), but a social disorder the witchdoctor demonstrates. Snake ribs are taken from the man's head - an image of unease, and hair, teeth and bones, matter out of place, are found by the family (not the witchdoctor) at the house entrance. The witchdoctor's compensation is fully adapted to his mystique. It is valuable farm animals, but of a colour (white, *mweu*) associated by the Kamba with brilliance and beauty. The witchdoctor reads the signs of disorder and provides remedies for that greater affliction.

The writer's confidence in this practitioner and his proceeding is based upon the certainty that the witchdoctor works on a spiritual plane that includes human affliction among its effects. His materials are appropriately outlandish: parts of the body where they do not belong and herbs instead of food. The witchdoctor sustains this confidence more by the powerful significance of his acts and symbols than by the pragmatic efficacy of his treatment.

The witchdoctor is not a "traditional healer", because there is no non-traditional healer to contrast with him. To have designated him into a category of traditional healers immediately simply sets up the terms of a contrast which did not exist before this category was described. The numerous types of healers that existed both within and among different cultural groups in what became Kenya are now absorbed into a single large category (Good, 1987) confronted by the contrasting techniques of biomedicine. "Tradition" then is used globally to refer to what was done before the advent of biomedicine and to what is opposed to biomedical procedure. Where no general system existed one is now generated by a set of opposing categories. Whereas biomedicine is scientific and experimental, traditional medicine is intuitive and received; and whereas biomedicine is Western in orientation traditional medicine is African. Traditional healing, crystalized from a complex mixture of transmitted and fabricated practices, stands against the formalities of biomedicine where in the past those practices existed with no reference at all to medicine or to each other.

Traditional Medicine Versus Biomedicine

When Elias began to experience serious intestinal blockage, he first gave thought to using herbal remedies. When a tea he had made of leaves failed to give him relief, he consulted an elderly woman in the locality known for her mastery of herbal medicine. She gave him a concoction, the ingredients of which she refused to reveal but which she said would work because of its "slippery" nature. Elias began to take this medicine, but before he could gauge its effect, his sons, both of whom worked as technicians at the hospital, insisted that he goes for surgery to remove the obstruction. He was finally persuaded to take the trip and to submit to the operation. The operation was a success. While he was recuperating, a group of his relatives, having heard of a rumour that he had died on the operating table, arrived at the hospital and started wailing before they were convinced that he had survived the operation.

In such a case as explained above, one chooses the more readily available, less expensive and less immediately risky remedy of the herbalist, starting with the usual resort of self-dosage but then consulting a local specialist. In great pain and eager for a cure, he is cajoled into submitting to the radical procedure of surgery by those connected with the medical establishment. Some of his other relatives interpret his submission (or his absence from home) as death and respond accordingly. Note that procedures are not abandoned, but are put aside in favour of others that seem to attack the problem more directly. There is an interplay of confidence. Elias trusts the herbal method, but his pain and the urging of his "modern" sons impel him towards the neo-medical solution, yet there is evidence that his relatives, however they might feel about herbal treatment, do not have complete confidence in the ability of the bio-medical procedure to save his life. In this case, a global treatment (like that of the Kamba witchdoctor) gives way to the much more specific treatment of the hospital. The local treatment is becoming traditional in being local, more readily accessible, personal and inexpensive, attributes which both encourage and discourage confidence, as do their opposites in biomedicine. The sons have confidence in biomedicine while Elias has to be persuaded to accept it. However, the relatives are not persuaded.

It is well known that biomedicine does not inspire full and complete confidence in respect to its treatment as well as practitioners– the invasive and impersonal nature of its treatment as well as its lack of emphasis on prevention can be as distressing as they are inspiring. It may not be surprising that those encountering biomedical treatment for the first time are dented in the same way as those who have had experience in it. The procedures that have become identified as traditional, the Kamba case notwithstanding, do not uniformly inspire trust in those who make use of them. There are doubts about traditional healing, and these doubts are different from those expressed in biomedicine.

Confidence in biomedicine has a different basis from confidence in local healing practices. The Luo sage Oruka Rang'inya (Odera Oruka, 1991:126) summarized the nature of this confidence in one type of healer, the *ajuoga,* in terms of a family situation. A child is sick, the wife insists that the healer must be called in. The husband complies and the child gets well vindicating the wife. Of course the child may not get well but Oruka Rang'inya does not consider the mechanics of the *ajuoga's* healing, but rather his ability to gain a psychological edge because of the constitution of the family.

> So we see these medicinemen have to be good and effective psychologists to justify their existence. They work by instilling confidence in the sick. A patient believes in his imminent recovery when the medicineman gives him the assurance that he will get better, and almost invariably the sick person does get better. This confidence is founded upon a false premise that because a medicineman is an authority in the art of curing the sick, whenever he speaks, he certainly cannot go wrong.

The medicineman creates confidence because the aura of confidence, which already surrounds him due to the repute of his powers, can itself effect a cure.

While the above pattern apparently operates with regard to medical doctors and others in their own home countries (with degree, titles and instruments taking the place of the medicineman's reputation), it cannot work for them where their techniques are unfamiliar and the institutions granting their degrees are unknown. They must rely upon the simple efficacy of the treatments and the (Christian) religious and educational institutions to lend them credence. It should be noted that the medicineman already has the institutional support for his work in the family, clan, village and other social forms. As the physician bases his claim to efficacy upon pragmatics, he can be tied to that claim when his cures fail. Confidence can be withheld and, if provisionally extended, can quickly be withdrawn when the surgery is not a success and the drugs do not save a life. The medicineman only fails if the family and other institutions refuse to or are unable to support him. Therefore, each kind of practitioner gains or loses confidence on the terms which have been set for him.

As biomedicine advances its claims, traditional healing builds opposition–biomedicine must base itself upon practical demonstration and outside authority. As in the above instance, Elias' sons have gone over to biomedicine as they have moved to careers outside agriculture and the village's social world. Elias is drawn into biomedical treatment by the external and medical factors. These factors constitute the internal and familial confidence. Many people continue to live in the world that the Kamba man and Oruka Rang'inya describe, but its conditions also change. Though both biomedicine and traditional healing practices have separate and distinct characteristics, they are both reformed by their encounter with each other. The resulting confidence (or lack of it) that each is accorded takes the shape of that encounter. However, this encounter is not symmetrical, whereby biomedicine exerts more pressure upon local healing practices than the vice versa. This owes to its association with urban, Western and politically and economically potent lifestyles and also perhaps due to successful cures.

Traditional healing therefore forms within a dialectic with biomedicine. While doing what biomedicine does not do, the traditional healer tries increasingly to do it in the same way. While appealing to the base of a local, familial confidence in his powers, he in effect tries to construct himself into the role of the family physician in European and American societies all the while maintaining an indigenous African claim to his parents' confidence.

This is, however, a speculation for which I have not yet produced evidence. I am in effect designing a model of confidence in traditional healing based upon two bodies of information that I have established; the existence of a variety of indigenous healing practitioners who derive their confidence from the repute their position in the community gives them, and the alien and challenging approach to biomedicine to these settings. The result, is the incipient fashion of a traditional healing which begins to encompass a variety of local practices both to oppose and emulate the science and system of biomedicine.

Biomedicine has its origins in the urbanizing, industrializing setting of the West. In its emergence it forced the existing 'folk' healing into opposition and emulation situation much as the capitalist economic system forced local markets and the barter exchange system to adopt its money operation and its patterns of accumulation. As biomedicine enforced scientific rigour in its concepts and in the training of its practitioners, it rejected numbers of notions and their advocates, mud-treatments and quicksilver and ginseng and magnetism. An array of herbal treatments became loosely organized under the rubric of homeopathy in opposition to biomedicine's allopathy. Chiropractic, the predecessor of the American homeopathy that emphasized conservative treatment, massage and preventive nutrition, had to organize itself like biomedicine to sustain confidence and for the chiropractors to be recognized as "doctors".

The ancient Indian system of Ayurveda has developed physician-like specialists who see their patients in hospitals of their own. Chinese acupuncturists and herbalists, despite the scientific validation of their techniques, are under increasing pressure from their government to conform to medical standards and appearance. This capacity of biomedicine to undermine and force less well-organized indigenous practices into systematic opposed conformity has been having its effects in Kenya.

In a survey of attitudes towards "traditional medical care" in Kingoti and Kambusu sub-locations of Machakos District, Van Luijk (Van Ginneken and Muller, 1988:304) found that "as a last resort in case of serious misfortunes or disease, a very high percentage of the inhabitants . . . would still go to *mundu mue*, but as there were so many "thresholds" and the price in money and social cost was so high, visits were relatively infrequent." Most of Van Luijk's 108 respondents said that Christians are not allowed to go to *mundu mue*, and a number stated that they would conceal such a visit because it might lead to disrepute and accusations of paganism. For these Kamba informants, confidence in the healers was overlaid by a need to avoid the communal disfavour that choosing a local healer would incur. Interestingly, none of them cared about being thought of as rejecting biomedical treatment by visiting a local healer. It is the religious implications of a visit to such a healer that concerned them greatly whereas they made regular visits to clinics without any such qualms.

In this and other similar bodies of statistical information (Mburu, 1974) about Kenya's healing choices, it is clear that the formative antagonism between traditional healing and biomedicine is not so plain to the people themselves as is the need to reject such 'pagan' practices and practitioners as urged by the Christian churches. This is another side of the dialectical break which helps to define what traditional healers are considered socially – they face modern medicine both as witchdoctors and as pagans, while biomedicine is both empirical and, by implication, Christian; after all it was the Christian missionaries who first made biomedical treatment and biomedical training available to Kenyans (Beck, 1974:91). Thus, it would seem that the only way to consult traditional healers would be on the sly, while running the risk of condemnation by the congregation as a wilful sinner. Apparently, open loyalty to traditional healing could only take the form of wholesale rejection of Western imports of biomedicine, Christianity, capitalism and the whole range of Western imports. This is the avenue some "traditionalist" groups have taken, according to research work undertaken by undergraduate students of Moi University.

To adopt such a global traditionalism (and anti-Western, anti-modernism) puts great pressure on traditional healing. Its practitioners themselves may not want to risk that extreme, but would prefer to be situated together with their patients in a "landscape of healing" or an "economy of therapy" such as that of the Luo of Siaya (Cohen and Odhiambo, 1988: 88-92) where people are not strongly oriented towards either traditional or biomedical practice, but are in search of both cures and opportunities to practice. The district hospitals, dispensaries and clinics are located in one place and have well-known attributes which qualify them within the whole system. Though the treatment is free of charge (immediately classifying them as a therapeutic population), it is also slow, grudging and, in the opinion of many, not of the right sort. Cohen and Odhiambo (1989) found that people in Siaya considered the health service practitioners not free enough given the alleged practice where they prescribe aspirin for everything. I discovered in Eldoret that people travel long distances (as did Elias) to wait for many hours for a doctor who might end up not seeing them and if he did, would probably send them for an unnecessary blood test or curtly issue a prescription.

Whereas biomedicine demands a sanitary environment, this prerequisite is not achieved in the hospitals or clinics. On the other hand, the instrumentality of drugs, tests and injections resembles more of the magical effects than science in action of which the traditional healers have been accused. Yet this may be due to lack of funding, lack of personnel or lack of training, so that economic conditions make biomedicine replicate the style and stance of traditional healing while maintaining its dignified rhetoric.

It should be noted that there are no two rigidly differentiated bodies of healing prowess facing each other in mortal competition. If traditional healing comes about and is like biomedicine due to imitation, biomedicine will be like traditional healing involuntarily and out of necessity. A man named Seringe, who trained as a medical assistant but left due to a serious car accident, told me two stories which define the actual scope of biomedical practice under these circumstances: There was a co-worker who regularly disappeared in the mornings after late nights away. He asked the man where he went and the man would reply that he used to visit the local dispensary for a morning-after penicillin shot to prevent him from contracting syphilis. One day, Seringe, knowing that syphilis cannot be prevented this way, went to the dispensary in the morning, broke through the groups of waiting men, and confronted the man. The assistant replied that he was poor and ill-paid for his work: He was earning ten shillings a shot and not causing any harm. If the men believed it might work then it might. In this case the medical assistant was behaving like the 'injection doctors' who ply their trade in many African countries (van der Geest, 1982), even at bus-stops in Kenya (McEvoy, 1976).

The other story is where Seringe urged the principal of the school to which he sent his children to require all the students to wear socks. Having seen the condition of the lavatories he feared the parasitic infections that barefoot children might pick up. The policy was instituted but Seringe found himself unable to afford socks for his own children. Subsequently, the principal sent the children home with the message that Seringe must be a hypocrite to require of others what he could not deliver himself. This indicates that biomedical knowledge bows to economic exigency and seems to become "traditional ignorance".

Indeed, the knowledge provided by biomedicine becomes agonizing in the absence of the capacity to act upon that knowledge. An item in the *Nation* Newspaper (22 July, 1992) reported that two people suffering from bites by a rabid dog in Kisii had gone for three days without receiving injections of anti-rabies vaccines because none could be found. It was after the two men travelled about the district seeking the vaccine that a single a dose was provided by a private clinic at Kshs. 1,400. Pasteur's triumphant discovery of the immunization principle was thus of little use to the two potential victims of rabies. This portrays the informal and heedless weakness of Western medicine; the failure to distribute it when urgently needed.

Confidence Building

As the substantive differences between biomedicine and traditional healing become blurred in the daily quest for health, it becomes important for practitioners to try to distinguish themselves by an appeal to the forms of both. Practitioners in both groups gain the confidence of those they propose to heal by taking the appearance of a healer people will recognize. Biomedical personnel can still assume the mantle of institutional medical authority however much their behaviour violates the laid down principles. Traditional healers on the other hand must seek a more delicate balance.

While biomedical personnel can always return to science and its institutional supports, traditional healers experience a double turn-around of the dialectic. Having already defined themselves in response to biomedicine, they must now redefine themselves in response to the mixed state of affairs where both category of practitioners tend to resemble; the traditional healer imitates the biomedical healer but only to a degree, never so much as to carry the liabilities of clinic and hospital medicine. His treatments, and even his personal aspect, become a hybrid of styles and devices and he incorporates whatever traditional healing forms are most recognizable as traditional. He at the same time borrows from a variety of different traditions while claiming a primary loyalty to one. This aims at seeking a broad clientele coming from varied distances and across ethnic boundaries for consultation while not alienating people of his own milieu – he acts as the doctor drawing those who need to think of him as *daktari* but no so much that he seems to be a doctor uninterested in such conditions as the failure at love and bad luck, which do not concern a medical doctor.

The arena of confidence in which the traditional healer operates is rather circumscribed; he has a wide range of options but he must array them carefully.* A model of confidence has emerged from these healers' self-fashioning in the wider world where they must confront, acknowledge and put aside biomedicine while retaining a connection with arcane, possibly invented, local practices. This model is visible in the most open expression of the healer's trade. For example, Morris Makini often advertises his 'natural remedies' in national newspapers and usually lists a set of towns and cities in Kenya that he hopes to visit in the coming month with precise places and times for consultation. He has a head office in Nairobi with telephone and fax numbers. However, his wide range of experience is in Tanzania. In his advertisements he sometimes includes testimonials as well as answers to questions of concern. In one of them he answered the question posed by Mrs. X of Nairobi:

* I deliberately use the pronoun "he" here because it is generally men who take up this level of traditional healing since women healers can still prosper at the local level. Moreover, the cosmopolitanism, which is an important symbolic attribute of the public traditional healer, seems to be more credible in men.

Question: What are the symptoms of Aids?

Answer: They are several, but most victims commonly complain of pains in the joints, stomach, chest and skin rashes, ulcers in the mouth, diarrhoea, loss of appetite, weight, hair, sweating, fatigue, numbness, general weakness and a chain of endless ailments.

Message: Aids virus knows no border. You can be a victim, mind your health and save your precious life. This is your only chance!!

This piece is followed immediately by: "Write enclosing a reply stamp to .... Dr. Morris Makini (address)"

Makini does not list AIDS among the diseases that he can remedy in the beginning of his advertisement. This question and answer piece is purely informational. Note that he fails to spell "AIDS" with uppercase letters, but does include authentic symptoms among his list. Although it is difficult to diagnose AIDS without a blood test, it opens up the possibility of anyone experiencing these varied symptoms to have AIDS. Nevertheless, he proposes AIDS as a disease within his purview, thus publicly bringing it within the realm of a "doctor" who neither claims to be medical in orientation, nor does he use the word "traditional" in his literature. He uses the word 'alternative', without stating explicitly what his remedies are in alternative to. Perhaps it is those with health and mental afflictions that he describes and traditional and biomedical healing might be the systems to which he provides the alternative. Whatever the content of his pharmacopoeia and the manner of his treatment, Makini has clearly established himself as a cosmopolitan, a medical doctor, a peripatetic and a traditional healer using herbal medications to treat scientifically named diseases yet safely enough without side effects.

Makini resembles, in a number of respects, the urban practitioners of Southeast Asia, South America and some parts of Africa, who have placed themselves between local tradition and international biomedicine, borrowing freely from each while quietly disavowing their unpleasant or dangerous aspects. Makini, like his colleagues elsewhere, needs to invent a device for suggesting that he can be trusted; despite the title "doctor" he lacks biomedical credentials and is equally unable to call upon the familial community references of the traditional healer. He seeks to develop confidence in the milieu of the newspaper (by no means anonymous or impersonal in Kenya) by calling up the artifacts which both biomedical and traditional healers employ. The potential patient who takes the initiative of writing to him or visiting him during his consultation hours approaches him with a confidence similar to that placed in a physical or traditional healer, but on his own terms. Apparently, Makini is inventing a kind of confidence appropriate to a healer for the urban masses who lack access to the other kinds of healers or who wish to be addressed in particular. He may be genetically related to the urban traditional healers as observed by Good and Kimani (1980) and Katz and Kimani (1982) whereby his evocation of biomedical forms is more subtle than the imitations and bare use of drugs practised by biomedical doctors.

Makini is not unique though his approach seems salient in some regards. Other traditional healers seek to define themselves in his manner vis-a-vis established healers, but also distinct from each other. The result, glimpsed through the public media and heard from sources on town streets, is a growing pluralism of healing that serves particular urban constituencies eclectically. There is, for instance, Shariff Omar Mohammed whose practice of magic and willingness to appeal to the spirits for the successful love life and business transactions of his customers seems a far cry from the herbalism of Makini. In the first place, he is drawing upon the labels of a Muslim confidence though he makes no reference to Islam in his newspaper advertisements, but offering to help as traditional healers were known to, dealing with personal issues that doctors and medical assistants do not consider. Yet his magic demands "utmost precise practice," like medical practice. However, in another advertisement he portrays himself less discrete than Makini, by making the rash claims of his "medicinal herbs from India and China with perfect curative effect on Aids related complex" plus a number of other diseases and symptoms. These symptoms include those of AIDS (weight loss and body weakness). On the contrary, Barton (1991:5), drawing upon an extensive survey of the anthropological and medical literature, attests that no one has recorded observations of traditional healers treating AIDS. Both Makini and Shariff do make it known that they are attentive to the disease and, as Milstein (1991) notes, the efforts of traditional healers to treat AIDS symptoms have at least won some support. On the other hand, the experience of Uganda, where AIDS nostrums have been hawked openly to hordes of buyers, should be viewed seriously.

It is very difficult to ascertain who actually consults these hybrid urban healers (hence, perhaps, Barton's conclusion). The actual confidence felt in their practices cannot be compared with the one they try to build. Hesitancy to admit visiting an urban healer may be congruent with the hesitancy of rural Christians to admit visiting a traditional healer. While the rural Christians use the pagan label for their secretiveness, urban dwellers are more likely to allege medical respectability (in respect of the healers). However, these eclectic urban practitioners have already anticipated this demureness and have therefore built reassurances in their advertisements and consultation settings.

This threat to confidence has caused some traditional healers seeking a wider and more urban clientele to move towards the adoption of more trappings of the physician. In a bid to develop the required confidence, Jack Githae, a herbalist with a wide local practice but no newspaper advertisement, first begàn by manufacturing and marketing his remedies, and then went on to initiate a formal training programme for future practitioners (see Chapter 5). Githae's Institute of Alternative Medicine and Technology, and which will accept its first class of students soon, is designed to pass on herbal medicine scientifically. In a printed interview (Mwakisha, 1992), Githae deplores the secretiveness of herbalists intent upon protecting their business and proposses an open training programme designed with the help of educators and staffed by qualified academics. Thus, in a stroke he hopes to eliminate the mystification surrounding herbalism and replace it with a publicly accredited and technically provable mastery of the medical properties of herbs. This rejects, the herbalists' traditional training and manner of practice while legitimizing the use of herbs. The herb, now known by a variety of local terminologies and used accordingly to special properties, will be known by a scientific name (e.g. *Datura stramonium*) with a specific pharmacology action.

National perspective

To innovators like Githae what is at stake is not only the capture of the urban and educated clientele that Makini is only tentatively luring, but also the introduction of Kenyan herbal medicine into the repertory of the national medical system. This can be seen as an extension of the "bonification" and the medical improvement of people and society that Beck (1974:104-105) sees as a basis for the "evolution of native society". The "professionalization" of herbalism that Githae and others are trying to bring about, parallel to a process generally occurring in traditional medicine throughout Africa (Last and Chavunduka, 1986), has the advantage of bringing traditional healing out of the social and religious conflict with biomedicine into the role it can play in a specific national medical system. It may also give herbalists access to educational facilities and funding already enjoyed by their would-be colleagues in biomedicine, besides making them eligible to collect fees from patients within the national health care system or from insurers. As a result, Kenyan herbalists are taking the path already taken by chiropractors in the United States, homeopaths in Britain, naturopaths in Germany, and Ayurvedic doctors in India, who are encountering the same obstacles.

In seeking to create a public confidence in traditional healing through biomedical procedures and training while retaining a more personal and local aspect, the reformed urban healers are also making themselves liable to a public reaction when their services fail to meet the expectations they have built.

With its colonial introduction biomedicine inherited a fixed position in the clinical and public health apparatus of the state. The licensing of health professionals and the provision of biomedical services both became government responsibilities in independent Kenya (Wisner, 1989: 68-83). Implicit in this alliance between the state and biomedicine is the relative immunity of biomedical personnel from legal recourse by disgruntled patients. The mammoth malpractice suits and consequent insurance fees that bedevil professional biomedicine in Europe and America are not so prominent in Kenya. Legal attention to biomedicine is mostly confined to government regulation under the supervision of the physicians themselves. Medical care is in such demand that objections to its manner and results are easily silenced. In effect confidence is enforced.

It should be noted that a similar situation existed with regard to traditional healers who relied upon the family and the local community to support them. There were established systems for recourse against them. However, studies of traditional medicine rarely provide information about conceptions of malpractice and error in treatment. Today traditional healers, and especially those who attempt to create public quasi-medical practices, are vulnerable to complaint. Their reputation is built in newspapers and by advertising rather than by kin advice or word of mouth. When their medicines fail or cause harm, their activity, especially if not legitimated by license and professionalism as in the case with biomedicine, can be redefined as criminal (i.e. whereas the failure of a doctor to live up to the confidence reposed in him is usually absorbed into the strictures of biomedicine, the failure of a traditional healer is regarded a crime because he has taken it upon himself to make claims which no system, whether local, social, international or scientific, will support). Thus, traditional healers, particularly those who venture outside their ethnic or local base, are in a zone of frail confidence.

Social perspective

Apparently, confidence in traditional healers is social in nature. The traditional healer whose procedures fail and having no context to excuse or to define his errors as an honest attempt to heal, has met no sympathy within the impersonal public realm. He is a criminal or a witch.

Mutungi (1977), while examining the legal aspects of witchcraft in East Africa, concludes that both witchcraft and medicine rely upon psychology and psychiatry for the efficacy of their treatments and that there is a lot to be gained from the recognition of the role of the witchdoctor in traditional African societies who has gained a mastery of such skills within the local context. This is the beneficial and open side of witchcraft, distinct from the dark malice of the sorcerer. In fact the same social system that supports and encourages the witchdoctor can equally form the accusation against harmful witchcraft. However, the skills of the witchdoctor might subject him to these accusations of harmful witchcraft. There are however, safeguards within those same social relations. The traditional healer who ventures outside these social relations and is not completely accepted into the biomedical system, might find the harmful sense of witchcraft applied to any exercise of his skills and in particular to any harm that might be blamed on him. The vagueness and pervasiveness of witchcraft accusations as an expression of disgruntlement merges with the law to create a particularly vulnerable specimen in anyone doing what the public traditional healer is trying to do. The promotion of confidence in traditional healers looks like biomedicine; breach of that confidence looks like witchcraft, which the state too has taken note of and is determined to define and regulate (Kenya, 1962). Here is a case in point.

Wambui visited Ndiru who advertises himself as a traditional healer and has an office in a nearby city. Wambui was seeking treatment for her inability to conceive. She had been unable to obtain any helpful advice from the medical assistant in her area or the doctor who saw her briefly at a clinic in the public hospital. Ndiru offered her treatment which he claimed would cause her husband's sperm to penetrate her eggs and make a child. The treatment was very expensive, but Wambui and her husband succeeded in raising the money from relatives. After a course of drinking preparations and performing exercises which Ndiru supervised, Wambui not only failed to conceive, but also fell sick. Her condition was diagnosed as an ulcer by the medical assistant. Those in Wambui's family who were aware of the treatment encouraged her to confront Ndiru with her problem and demand her money back, but Ndiru tried to persuade her that her condition was due to her failure to follow his instructions. She told her family that she was convinced Ndiru had caused her stomach problem because she refused to give him more money. The family sent a local elder to the doctor but he was unsuccessful in obtaining a refund. They then decided that they must either ask a politician to force the doctor to comply i.e. return the money and heal Wambui's ulcer, or find someone able to sue him in the High Court for damages. Their deliberations on this matter focused on the idea that Ndiru had caused Wambui's illness because she did not pay him enough, less on the doctor's failure to make her conceive.

Wambui's case might have gone on concurrently with the work of the Kamba witchdoctor described at the beginning of this chapter. The distance between these two forms of traditional healing is measured by the kind of confidence reposed in each. In the Kamba case, this confidence may have been complex and dialectical but it has been integrated so completely into the sense of belonging to the group that neither it nor its breach are visible in the group members' account.

Wambui goes to Ndiru because she finds no solution to her problem neither within the context that the witchdoctor occupies, nor within public medical facilities. She may have been crossing boundaries to find a new treatment, as has always been done, but she finds a treatment that fails and chooses to identify a coincident injury with the healer's malice though not primarily with his failed treatment. These two cases exist in the present Kenyan traditional medicine, which in one becomes the present of Kenyan civil authority as well. The healer has become the alien, afflicting presence previously represented by the jealous neighbours and the witch they employ.

REFERENCES

Barton, Thomas G. 1991. *Sexuality and Health in Sub-Saharan Africa: An Annotated Bibliography*. Nairobi: AMREF.

Beck, A. 1974. "History of Medicine and Health Services in Kenya (1900-1950); In *Health and Disease in Kenya* edited by L.C. Vogel et. al. Nairobi: East African Literature Bureau. pp. 91-106.

Carman, J. 1976. *A Medical History of the Colony and Protectorate of Kenya: A Personal Memoir*. London: Rex Collins.

Cohen, D. W. and E. S. Atieno-Odhiambo. 1989. *Siaya: The Historical Anthropology of an African Landscape*. Nairobi: Heinemann Kenya.

Good, C. M. 1987. *Ethnomedical Systems in Africa: Patterns of Traditional Medicine in Rural and Urban Kenya*. New York: The Guilford Press.

Good, C. M. and V. N. Kimani. 1980. "Urban Traditional Medicine: A Nairobi Case Study". *East African Medical Journal* 57, 5 (May): 301-316.

Katz, S. S., S. H. Katz and V. N. Kimani. 1982. "The Making of an Urban Mganga: New Trends in Traditional Medicine in Urban Kenya." *Medical Anthropology* 6, 2 (Spring): 91-112.

Kenya, Republic of. 1962. Witchcraft Act, Cap 67 *Laws of Kenya*.

Kleinman, A. 1978. "What Kind of Model for the Anthropology of Medical Systems? *American Anthropologist* 80 No. 3 (September): 661:665.

Last, M. and G. L. Chavunduka. 1986. *The Professionalisation of African Medicine*. Manchester: Manchester University Press.

Mburu, F. M. 1974. *Traditional and Modern Medicine Among the Akamba Ethnic Group of Upland Machakos, Kenya*. M.A. Thesis. Makerere University.

McEvoy, J. 1976. "The Bus-stop Dispenser" *East African Medical Journal* 53, 3 (March): 193-195.

Miller, N. and R. C. Rockwell. 1988. *AIDS in Africa: The Social and Policy Impact.* Lewiston, N.Y: The Edwin Mellen Press.

Milstein, M. H. 1991. "A Search in the Past to Cure a Modern Pestilence." *Daily Nation* 11th October, p. 3.

Mutungi, O. 1977. *The Legal Aspects of Witchcraft in East Africa: With Particular Reference to Kenya.* Nairobi: East African Literature Bureau.

Mwakisha, J. 1992. "Herbalist Embarks cn a Novel Project". *The Nation* 1 July p. 1.

Ndirangu, S. 1982. *A History of Nursing in Kenya.* Nairobi: Kenya Literature Bureau.

Odera, H. O. ed. 1991. *Sage Philosophy: Indigenous Thinkers and Debate on African Philosophy.* Nairobi: ACTS Press.

Van der Geest, S. 1982. "The Illegal Distribution of Western Medicine in Developing Countries: Pharmacists, Drug Peddlers, Injection Doctors and Others: A Bibliographic Exploration." *Medical Anthropology* 6,2 (Fall): 197-219.

Van Ginneken, J. K. and A. S. Muller, eds. 1984. *Maternal and Child Health in Rural Kenya: An Epidemiological Study.* London: Croom Helm.

Weisz, J. R. 1974. "East African Medical Attitudes" *Social Science and Medicine* 6:323-334.

Wisner, B. 1989. *Power and Need in Africa.* Trenton, NJ: Africa World Press.

Chapter 5

ETHONOMEDICAL PRACTICE IN KENYA The Case of the Karati Rural Service Centre

Jack K. Githae

Background

The Karati Rural Service Centre (KRSC) aims at serving rural communities in Kenya by applying the concept of appropriate technology. The Centre is geared towards the provision of simple industrial, agricultural, educational and health services to communities which find it difficult, even expensive, to seek such services from other institutions. By using appropriate technology, the Centre is able to tap the available resources for the benefit of the local population. In this way, the population served by the Centre develops a sense of exploiting the resources available in their own environment, using simple technologies that they can afford and whatever materials that are available to improve their lives.

The aim is to achieve wholesome development of the individual and the society as a whole. For example, by using readily available hoes and *pangas*, soils and trees, plus their own labour, people can put up a cheap but decent brick and timber building. From a health perspective, such a house may be more suitable as it is likely to keep warm and free from dust as opposed to a poor mud structure or an expensive modern stone building.

Our herbal practice is born of this philosophy; that we can use our local environment to meet most of our social, educational and health requirements. The medicines we make and dispense are thus the product of our local trees and vegetation.

Advantages of Herbal Medicine

To the individual patient herbal medicines have greater advantage than conventional medicines (i.e. pharmaceutical drugs). They are cheaper and more readily available and since they are natural, they tend to be less toxic–they do not have the toxic preservatives, binder and dyes that characterize most biomedicines. Herbal medicines are also wholesome, so that, besides controlling or curing illness, they provide the body with nutrients such as carbohydrates, proteins, minerals, vitamins and hormones that are required in times of sickness to speed up recovery.

Concentrating on treating the symptoms rather than a living organic system and the actual cause of disease, the administrators of biomedicine treat the body as if it were made up of many different individual and independent parts. As such, the efficacy of these drugs has been challenged by a number of indigenous communities; African herbalists have shown that their traditional methods of curing the sick are quite effective.

Herbal Medicine and Society

Mother nature in her eco-wisdom provided every part of the world with herbs that constitute appropriate cure for diseases most prevalent in the respective ecological set-up if appropriately studied, preserved, propagated and utilized. In our work, we have noted that wild animals, and to some extent domestic animals, in their natural settings instinctively treat themselves when they fall sick by consuming various parts of medicinal plants such as leaves, stems, barks and roots, which they dig up to get the right medicine. They may also vigorously rub themselves against appropriate plants with curative properties to treat their skin conditions. It is only when placed in an artificial set-up that they lose these instincts thereby becoming less adapted.

It is important to remember that human beings as well as animals have depended on herbs for food and medicines since time immemorial. Many species of medicinal plants of the world are known to have been used for food, treatment, prevention and cure of various diseases as well as in keeping men and women healthy. For example, according to the Holy Bible, Moses is reported to have prayed earnestly to the Lord who showed him a piece of wood which he threw into the water to make it fit for drinking (Exodus 17: 22-25). The Bible is indeed full of praises for herbs, encouraging man to take them without fear as they are God's provisions to him. God created herbal medicines out of the earth and hence a rational person will not hesitate to use them.

Nevertheless, human fascination with the exotic led him to believe that chemotherapy was a more effective and noble way of treating/curing the sick than herbal medicines. Thus, for the past 500 years, he has depended on isolated chemicals to cure his maladies. It should be noted that Hippocrates, that Greek doctor and father of modern medicine, was a herbal practitioner as were other famous doctors of the ancient times such as Pliny, St. Luke and Galen.

The Karati Rural Service Centre (KRSC)

KRSC work began at Karati in South Kinangop near Naivasha in 1974. Then a clinic was opened in Doonholm shopping centre in Nairobi and Nyahururu town in 1984. Later, new clinics were opened in Nyeri in 1987 and in Meru and Kericho in 1988 (Table 5.1). The opening of the branches made it possible for the Centre to take services closer to the clientele.

The KRSC specializes in herbal medicines for both humans and livestock and offers consultancy services in agricultural and livestock management. My herbal practice began while I was working as an agricultural extension officer in the mid-1970s. During my visits to the newly settled farmers in Nyandarua District, I realized that the people I was serving had serious problems of health and poverty. Whatever I was expected to do (i.e. carry out extension work) tended to be secondary as the people's quest for improved health took priority. Not being in a position to help all of them financially, I resorted to sharing my traditional healing skills acquired from my grandmother.

Table 5.1: KRSC patient attendance, 1984-90

Years	1984-1985			1987-1988			1989-1990		
Clinic	Male	Female	Total	Male	Female	Total	Male	Female	Total
Nairobi	1878	2491	4369	789	1102	1891	–	–	914
Nyeri	–	–	–	1303	959	2262	–	–	748
Meru	–	–	–	200	350	550	–	–	430
Nyahururu	450	553	1003	250	370	620	–	–	597
Kinangop	1566	1867	3433	518	572	1090	–	–	437
Kericho	–	–	–	520	550	1070	–	–	600
Total			8805			7483			3726

Note: Each of the clinics was operated once a week.

As more and more of these farmers got treated and cured, they passed word around and within a short time, I was forced to offer herbal therapeutic service every weekend to a great number of people. Before long, the weekend proved to be too short a time to attend to all the patients. Consequently, I switched from a part-time herbal practitioner to a full-time one in 1982. During the initial stages of my practice, patients would voluntarily bring water and fire wood with them to be used in the preparation of the medicine. The Centre's clientele grew and the demand for these services extended beyond Kinangop to other parts of Kenya. Then I introduced a processing fee for patients. The fee was the same for every patient regardless of the nature and stage of illness.

Ethnomedical practice

Ethnomedicine refers to medical practice based largely or entirely on a localized scale and to people of a specific ethnic background. A cursory look at the distribution and background of the clientele seeking medical attention at KRSC clearly shows that traditional medicine is widely patronized. Those seeking assistance from KRSC come from all parts of the country as do herbal materials from which our medicines are extracted and prepared (Table 5.2). Between July 1989 and June 1990, some 18,720 patients were treated at our clinics countrywide. The clientele appears to represent the Kenyan population in respect to ethnicity, age, sex, professions and socio-economic status.

Table 5.2: Origin of patients to KRSC attendance per district by gender

District	Male	Female	Total
Nyeri	670	860	1530
Nairobi	510	560	1070
Kiambu	280	340	620
Murang'a	185	270	455
Nakuru	120	130	250
Nyandarua	70	90	160
Laikipia	40	60	100
Embu	40	50	90
Meru	20	30	50
Machakos	15	20	35
Narok	10	20	30
Mombasa	20	18	38
Kericho	15	35	50
Others	90	210	300
Total	2085	2695	4778

Diseases treated

Out of the 18,720 patients from all over the country, some 20 per cent complained of illnesses related to the nervous system, for example, paralysis and epilespy. Fourteen per cent complained of diseases related to the respiratory system including asthma, bronchitis and pneumonia, while some 13 per cent complained of various abdominal problems such as diarrhoea, dysentery, gastric/duodenal ulcers and constipation. Eleven per cent complained of bone and joint diseases such as rheumatism and arthritis. (Herbs are fairly effective and have no residual effects on the already weak joints and offer speedy recovery). Another 11 per cent complained of cardio-vascular problems most of whom appeared to have come from urban areas – herbs are especially effective in nourishing and replenishing the heart and surrounding blood vessels giving these organs the impetus required to perform their functions properly. For example we have had cases of very high blood pressure, 250/160, and on administering our herbal formulations for a week the blood pressure would drop to 150/130.

While response to herbal treatment has been excellent for all the above conditions, those who come to us with liver and spleen conditions, including diabetes, have by far recorded the quickest and the best results. Over 8 per cent of the patients who came with confirmed cases of diabetes from hospital got better within a short time provided they rigorously followed the dietary regime that was prescribed.

Sources of Drugs

The herbal medicines that we use are wholesome in that they provide a cure and nutrients to the individual to keep him/her healthy even after recovery. The source of these medicines is almost exclusively plant material. We harvest leaves, bark, roots and seeds of wild plants. Most of our medicines are obtained from the roots as shown in Table 5.3. Since destroying the roots results in the death of the whole plant, research in medicinal plants is being carried out to help identify chemical components in the other parts of the plants to see if, for example, leaves could be substituted for roots so as to help conserve plants (see Chapter 13).

Of the medicinal plants that we collect, we normally take note of the conditions which they treat, the part that is used and the popularity score of each of them. We have noted that one plant can treat more than one condition and several plants can treat one condition. It should, therefore, be possible to establish a standard herbal formula for a given condition in future.

Table 5.3 Percentage contribution of various plant parts to herbal medicines

Part	Percentage
Leaves	20
Roots	35.5
Whole Plant	20.0
Stem/Bark	8.0
Fruit	5.5
Seeds	3.0
Stem	3.0
Tubers	2.0
Flowers	2.0
Bulbs	1.0
Others	2.5

Processing of herbal medicines

During the formative years of KRSC, we used to chop pieces of plants which were then boiled and the resulting liquid put in jerrycans for dispensing. However, as the medicines were stored with no preservatives, they would get spoilt after a short time. As a result it was thought that if these medicines were stored and dispensed in powder form, then they would last longer. Thus KRSC adopted this new processing method.

Now at KRSC the processing of herbal medicines involves wholesome harvesting and collecting of raw plant materials, hygienic drying, grinding, mixing (according to specific drug formulae), packaging and storage. This is a demanding and expensive exercise which requires well trained personnel, especially in the fields of identification of medicinal plants, for collection and specific drug formulation. For harvesting and collection, intensive work is necessary.

Herbal medicine and modern technology

Over the years we have been of the opinion that it is only by continually studying and carrying out research in herbal medicine that we can hope to succeed and continue to offer improved services. We discovered from the very outset that without establishing the scientific basis and explanation for our drug formulae, treatment and analysis, we would not be able to offer credible services in an advancing technological environment in which scientific explanations to issues are being sought all the time.

It is with this understanding that, despite the staggering costs involved, we have endeavoured to acquire some modern and advanced equipment in herbal analysis such as a gas liquid chromatography machine for identification of chemical components of the plants used for medicine, a computer for purposes of storing and analyzing patient information, and a clinical analyzer (Reflotron machine) used in clinical chemistry analysis. Other equipment like glucometre and the stethoscope have not been ignored in the herbal practice at the KRSC.

When most patients come to our clinics, they often wonder whether we really are traditional-cum-herbal practitioners or modern conventional medical practitioners because of our use of modern techniques in diagnosis and treatment. This is because as people who have a lot of faith in science, we do not shy away from using any new technology that would prove useful to our practice and upgrade herbal medicines.

General response to herbal therapy

As indicated earlier in this chapter, traditional healing, including herbal practice has often been associated with witchcraft, sorcery and primitive divination. However, being a herbalist I have had a number of experiences with a number of people of different backgrounds through whom I have been in a position to learn a lot as well as assess their stands as far as herbal medicines are concerned.

Patients

In my clinics I receive patients of three main categories: The first group comprises those who come to the clinic because they regard herbal clinics as any other clinics. They are normally sure of recovery. We encounter no problems with this group and when the patients take our medicine, it does not take long before they recover and can do without further medication.

The second group is made up of those patients who come to try and see whether herbal medicines truly work, especially having failed to get well after consulting a few biomedical doctors. Some, even after deciding to come to see us, are still skeptical about herbal medicines while others expect miraculous recovery despite the fact that it might have taken them long with biomedical doctors. However, those who, although still doubtful, agree to take our prescriptions as instructed are amazed at the speed of recovery. This is the group that has earned us a lot of popularity by telling how they were cured of an "impossible" condition.

The third group, which forms most of our patients, come to us as a last resort.

They are desperate people who have tried many hospitals and doctors in vain. Some patients respond very well to our medication, especially those suffering from diabetes, cardio-vascular and respiratory conditions, depending on the nature and stage of the disease. Other patients, especially those with advanced cancer cases, take long to show positive response (i.e. if they adhere strictly to the medication). Most of them, being desperate individuals, cooperate as far as prolonged medication is concerned.

Research scientists

Quite a number of researchers come to us out of curiosity. They want to see whether what we do is really of any scientific value. They are not biased and, on seeing our scientific approach to herbal medicines, they get fascinated and become serious supporters of them and in due course assist where necessary. These researchers include biochemists, botanists and agriculturalists.

Other researchers are postgraduate students gathering information for their own research work. Some never come back after getting what they were looking for; others become even more interested in the information I give give and come back, this time not to gather information but to work with us to upgrade herbal medicine in Kenya.

Another group is composed of colleagues and relatives who try to support us in every possible way. They are quite enthusiastic in the promotion of herbal medicines to the highest standard possible.

The last group is made up of critics. Criticism is good because it presents a challenge to us and makes us tackle herbal medicines scientifically so that at the end of it all we have some data and analytical findings to present if need be to support our work.

University trained clinicians

In my work, I have not ignored university trained clinicians as they would be of great help in the diagnosis of diseases. At KRSC we have over the years endeavoured to improve relations between conventionally trained clinicians and ourselves because we realize that we have a common objective: saving the lives of our people and improving their health. Some of these clinicians are our patients, while others are our friends. They have a very positive attitude towards us and we work very closely as they help us by guiding and campaigning for us. Others are some of our patients' personal doctors who refer their patients to us and, on treating them successfully for cases such as diabetes, hypertension and epilepsy, they build trust in us and keep referring more patients to the Centre.

Another group comprises admirers and genuine supporters. These have even gone to an extent of offering to work with us part-time, and a few joined us on full-time basis.

In spite of the few problems we have encountered with a few clinicians, there is high hope that conventional medicine will one day intermarry with herbal medicine so that we can help humanity fully and effectively.

We have incorporated a number of full- time as well as part-time professionals in our undertakings. They include a specialist in the analysis of chemical components of various herbs using the gas liquid chromatography machine, who also assists in the encapsulation of our herbal medicines for use by some of our patients abroad; and a data analysis consultant (he is currently pursuing a Ph.D in mathematics at Harvard University) handling all data at KRSC. Others are; two trained clinicians in charge of clinical work; a forester responsible for herbal nurseries and agromedical gardens; a botanist responsible for identification of herbal plants; a senior clinical laboratory technologist working in conjunction with a trainee at the Kenya Polytechnic; and, a biochemist pursuing a Ph.D degree at the University of Nairobi.

Government and Herbal Therapy

As a herbalist, I must say that I have been quite impressed by the government's positive response towards herbal medical practice. This is evident in the Ministry of Health's proposal to have herbalists trained occasionally at the Kenyatta National Hospital on how to attend to their patients. Moreover, when the dreaded AIDS came up, the ministry did not hesitate to call on the herbalists to join them in search of a treatment for the disease. However, herbalists lack a statutory provision to safeguard/protect them. I therefore appeal to the government to facilitate the formulation of such an Act endorsing the protection of herbalists. For herbal therapy to work and be more beneficial to the human race, it should have the total support of patients, scientific researchers, university trained clinicians and the government. I appeal to all those concerned to arise and let us embark on improving herbal medicine for our own good today and in future.

Chapter 6

MANAGING ILLNESS AMONG THE LUO*

Isaac Sindiga

The health systems available in Kenya range from biomedical (Western) facilities, African traditional medicine and foreign traditional medicine such as Unani, Ayurveda and acupuncture, to certain transitional forms such as unqualified dispensers of modern drugs (see Chapter 1). These medical systems co-exist and may complement or compete with one another (Fabrega, 1982; Chapter 3). Thus, medical pluralism continues to be a reality in Kenya despite government encouragement and development of only the biomedical system.

Medical pluralism is significant in area of decision-making with regard to seeking and selecting therapy (as seen in Chapter 2). Many African communities categorize disease and illness according to cause. This in turn may influence therapy-seeking and selecting behaviour. Patients will go to biomedical facilities when their families, friends or neighbours, or even themselves, believe that an illness is naturalistic – they will turn to traditional healers when they conceive an illness to be caused by human–induced forces. However, when faced with actual illness, patients in the African context have been observed to be quite flexible, sometimes using a number of systems together for the same episode of illness (Ampofo and Johnson–Romauld, 1978; Mbiti, 1969).

This chapter examines the influence of a group's concept of disease causation on actual therapy-selecting behaviour within an environment of pluralism. Using the case of the Luo-speaking people of South Nyanza District, it is demonstrated that, although disease aetiologies are articulated, this does not lead to clear-cut selection of a medical system when faced with actual sickness. The chapter suggests a possible explanation for this variance. The following is an outline of the disease aetiologies upon which background the therapy-seeking behaviour is

---

* The data reported in this chapter were collected with financial support from the International Development Research Centre and the Rockefeller Foundation of New York. The funding is gratefully acknowledged.

discussed. This is done by offering field data from a client-based inquiry at the homes of traditional healers.

Study Area

Surrounding the Kenyan side of Lake Victoria are the Luo-speaking River-Lake Nilotes who occupy the three districts of Siaya, Kisumu and South Nyanza.* These Nilotes originated in the Bahr el Ghazal area in the Sudan around AD 1300 and migrated southwards through Uganda.

South Nyanza is an under-developed district with an estimated population of 1,305,000 in 1990 (Kenya, 1989:10). Eighty-five per cent of the population comprises the Luo. In this District health conditions are poor and life expectancy at birth is 49 years compared to a national average of 63 years (Kenya, 1989:137). This shows significant improvement from an estimated 34.6 years in 1969 (Sindiga, 1985). The crude death rate is 19 per 1000 with the major causes of mortality (according to hospital data) being: anaemia which accounts for 37 per cent of the total; malaria, 19 per cent; diarrhoea, 15 per cent; intestinal diseases, 9 per cent; and measles, 7 per cent (Odada and Otieno, 1990). (Malaria is endemic in South Nyanza.) Other common causes of morbidity are schistosomiasis, skin disease and sleeping sickness.

The infant mortality rate is 130 per 1000 live births compared to the national average of 80 per 1000 live births. About a decade ago, the District had a mortality rate of 266 per 1000 live births for those under five years (Kenya, n.d: 92). In 1990, the infant and child death rate was more than 216 per 1000 live births compared to a national average of 125 per 1000 (Odada and Otieno, 1990).

Despite the bleak health record, South Nyanza is poorly served with health facilities. As such, most people do not have to choose between traditional medicine and the modern one.

Luo Disease Aetiologies

Contrary to the impression created by earlier studies that, in Africa, diseases are believed primarily to come from supernatural causes (Yoder, 1982: 11-12), recent empirical work shows multiple causes. The Luo believe that disease and illness may be caused through at least five ways; diseases of the air, water and food; diseases caused by humans; diseases of the "living dead"; diseases of inheritance;

* South Nyanza has since been subdivided into three districts, namely, Homa Bay, Migori and Kuria districts; Luo-speakers live in Homa Bay and Migori districts.

and, diseases resulting from breaching taboos or customs. I will discuss each of these causes in turn.

Air, water and food

The Luo recognize that disease and illness may come from "bad" air – involving seasonal changes in weather and wind patterns. Weather usually changes from wet to dry, cold to hot, and vice versa and these changes are held to cause certain diseases such as flu and common cold. Malaria, which is associated with mosquitoes, is common in the rainy season. Drinking dirty water and eating contaminated food may also lead to such problems as abdominal pains, dysentery and typhoid. Contaminated food may cause diarrhoea (*diep*) which in turn may induce headache (*wich bar*).

Also, poor diet and food shortage, especially among infants and children, may cause diseases like marasmus and/or kwashiorkor (*hero*). This problem reflects poor weaning practices.

Finally, winds blowing from one place to another may carry along disease-causing bacteria. Boils (*yamo*) are believed to come about in this way and may also be caused by seasonal changes in wind patterns. Diseases in this category are sometimes called naturalistic diseases of God (Foster, 1976).

Human-caused disease

Within the second disease aetiology, the Luo recognize that evil people within a community may direct harm to their enemies or adversaries using sorcery and witchcraft. Sorcery (*nawi*) involves a situation where a sorcerer (*janawi*) applies his medicine to harm someone. Usually, the *janawi* grows certain herbs whereby when the seeds germinate, the target person begins to get ill. The herbs may also be ground into powder and buried under the doorstep, off the gate or in the house of the target person where it generates illness (Ocholla-Ayayo, 197:157).

Luo witchcraft may be inborn, inherited or acquired by undergoing special ceremonies and rites (Ocholla-Ayayo, 1976). The *janawi* appears to be the most feared person in the world of Luo medicine as he uses extremely potent materials to cause harm. In the words of Ocholla-Ayayo (1976:156-157), "*nawi* is a powerful destructive offensive medicine . . . *Nawi* contains some of the most poisonous plants and other minerals known . . ." such as crocodile gall juice. Nevertheless, *janawi* can also treat cases of *nawi*; in this capacity he works for the good of society and is called *jahoso*.

Certain witches use special herbs and other medicines to cause illness. The witches (*jondagla*–sing. *jandagla*) stuff their medicine (*ndagla*) into certain material objects, say dead snakes, rats, birds, chicken or rotten eggs, and place these either in the farm or along the pathway to the home of the target person. Once the latter crosses the object, he/she becomes ill immediately. Also, the Luo believe that witches (*jojuok,* sing, *jajuok*) can send a fly directly into a person's mouth. Upon swallowing, the fly settles in the lungs from where it begins to generate infections such as chest pains (*kor maremo*) and coughing (*ahonda*).

Another form of witchcraft is what the Luo call *juok wang* (evil eye) which is possessed by certain individuals who stare at their target individuals especially while eating. The food in the victim's stomach turns poisonous and causes abdominal pain and constipation. *Juok wang* tends to be transmitted by women and may be inherited by daughters through the force of evil spirits (*juogi*). Most of its victims are children.

The living dead

Disease among the Luo may also be caused by the supernatural. Each living family is obligated to keep and lubricate vertical relationships between itself and the living dead (See also Chapters 9-11 on the Abagusii, Abaluyia and Kikuyu).

The notion of maintaining and lubricating the vertical relationships is based on the view that the living dead are closer to God by virtue of their physical departure from the earth and can, therefore, intercede quite successfully between the living within their lineages and God (Mbiti, 1969). If the living ignore lubricating the relationships, then the living dead refuse to pray for the living to God and will show their anger by causing disease, illness and misfortune. Among the traditional Luo diseases "was the sanction to force the living to maintain proper relations with the dead" (Whisson, 1974:286).

Sometimes, spirits (*juogi*) of the living dead may, via dreams and/or illness, make certain demands on the living. For example, if one of the departed family members was a traditional healer (*ajuoga*), his/her spirits may demand that a certain surviving member of the lineage takes up his or her vocation. Should this revelation be ignored, then the ancestor will send the message forcefully by inducing disease such as mental disturbance (*neko*).

Disease inheritance

Yet there are certain diseases which appear to be inherited. The Luo believe that certain diseases such as epilepsy (*ndulue* or *ndulume*) and some mental disturbances are genetically perpetuated through offsprings.

Breach of taboos and customs

Finally, the Luo believe that breaching taboos or customs results in illness and misfortune to the offending person or his family. The most talked about consequence of breaching taboos is what is called *chira*, literally the wasting away of the body ultimately leading to death. Contrary to some scholars who associate the condition with malnutrition (e.g. K'Okul, 1991) or AIDS, (Acquired Immune Deficiency Syndrome), *chira* is a sin-consequence for breaching a taboo or custom (Ocholla-Ayayo, 1976).

Chira may manifest itself through certain diseases such as headache, coughing and diarrhoea, conditions which persist and cause progressive loss of weight. Other consequences of *chira* are infertility, giving birth to children of only one sex, children dying after birth, and children contracting incurable diseases (Ocholla-Ayayo, 1976:106). Conditions caused by *chira* are said to be incurable through modern medicine. This phenomenon appears to be part of the social and moral control on family and lineage life. It governs a wide array of aspects of everyday activities ranging from sexual propriety to communal life.

Luo Therapy-Seeking Behaviour

A group's disease aetiologies will influence therapy-seeking and selecting behaviour (see Chapter 2). It would appear that if the cause of a given episode of illness is taken to be naturalistic, then the patient (and his/her relatives) will seek therapy in modern medicine. Conversely, if an illness is believed to be human-induced, then therapy will be sought in traditional medicine. The Luo believe that Western medicine is ineffective for disease for which causes are human-related, but is taken to be efficacious in natural diseases which have their origins in environmental circumstances. Traditional medicine deals with both.

In this chapter, I set to argue that the fact that the Luo may and do distinguish multiple disease aetiologies notwithstanding, therapy-seeking behaviour does not always follow this distinction. People move freely from one medical system to another even on the same episode of illness. This appears to be caused partly by the confusion caused by the diffuse nature of symptoms; patients and their relatives and/or friends seek therapy in both traditional medicine and modern medicine because of the difficulties of interpreting symptoms and determining the cause of a given episode of illness. Other factors are nevertheless pertinent and include educational background and religious affiliation.

Also, any one disease may not be caused exclusively in one way. Moreover, a disease caused in a naturalistic manner may at another episode be human-induced as the symptoms tend to be similar. For example, headache and fever are clear signs of malaria but the same symptoms may be brought by *ndagla* and/or *nawi*. Likewise mental illness (*neko*) may be human-induced, inherited or a result of breaching a taboo, while marasmus can be caused by insufficient or poor quality food though the progressive wasting away and general poor health of an infant could come about as a result of breaching a taboo or custom.

The Luo recognize that certain diseases, say tuberculosis, asthma and malaria, are efficiently treated and cured by biomedicine. However, as already stated above, the inability to know the underlying cause of a disease makes people go to a health facility and at the same time turn to traditional healers. The idea is to seal any conflicting symptoms and maximize on recovery. Another common practice is to go to a health facility to forestall the progress of a disease and this gives time to the patient and his/her relatives to go to a traditional healer (*ajuoga*) to identify the cause of a particular illness by giving *manyasi*, a herbal concoction intended to identify the underlying cause of a disease (Table 6.1). Another way of identifying the cause of an illness is through divination which may be done by a *jalek* (seer, dreamer), *jakoro* (diviner), *jaulo* (spiritualist) or *jabilo* (fortune teller).

Table 6.1: Major categories of Luo traditional healers*

Category		Functions
Singular	*Plural*	
ajuoga	ajuoge	traditional healer (general)
yadh nyaluo	joyadh nyaluo	herbalist
jakoro	jokoro	diviner
jalek	jolek	seer, dreamer
jachomo	jochomo	bone-setter, physiotherapist
jangad lim	jongad lim	surgeon - extracts teeth; removes epiglottis
jaulo	joulo	spiritualist
nyamrerwa	nyamreche	traditional birth attendant. The term also connotes one's doctor, counselor, etc.
jatak	jotak	person who makes an incision into the stomach using a small horn (tum) to suck out undigested food which may result from constipation or evil eye (juok wang).
jabilo	jobilo	magician, fortune teller

SOURCE: Own field work, 1989

* An individual may combine one or more of these categories. *Jachomo*, for example, must necessarily possess knowledge of herbs which she/he uses in the work.

*Why patients go for traditional medicine**

In order to understand therapy-seeking behaviour among the Luo, I conducted a client-based inquiry at the homes of traditional healers. The strategy was to interview in detail and observe patients who were found consulting a number of traditional healers. Using case histories, I sought to establish certain principles: Why do patients go to see traditional healers? What are the profiles of the patients who seek traditional medicine? How do they make choices of therapy? Who makes such decisions? And what are the patterns of consultation of the various medical systems? (This included the reasons for consulting a traditional healer, whether this was a first visit for the current episode of illness, and whether the patient had earlier visited another, different, traditional healer and/or health facility.)

The field investigation approach in Ndhiwa Division of Homa Bay District involved interviews with clients of traditional healers using a semi-structured interview schedule rather than a prepared questionnaire. I found that consumers of traditional medicine are both men and women of various social and economic backgrounds, who span different age groups and profess various religious backgrounds. The following capsules will demonstrate this and the course of therapy-seeking as well as illuminate the way therapy-choices are made.

Case 1: Mary

My research team caught up with Mary at the home of a traditional birth attendant (TBA) at Rapedhi Village, Kanyikela Sub-location, Kanyidoto Location of Ndhiwa Division during the afternoon of September 18, 1989. The TBA had just delivered Mary's baby girl, her first child. Mary, aged 20 and whose home was at Gem in Rangwe Division, was an untrained primary school teacher at Olale in Ndhiwa. She had completed her Advanced Level Education at Segenge Girls High School in neighbouring Kisii District in 1988. At the time of the interview, she was a member of the Full Gospel Church having given up her affiliation to the Christian Church in Africa. She had been "admitted" at the TBA's home the previous day, September 17, 1989, after she came for an antenatal check-up with the TBA but developed labour and delivered her baby that night.

This was not Mary's first visit to the TBA's home. She had developed lower abdominal pains when she was 5 months into the pregnancy. She could not walk properly, nor could she sit for any prolonged period. She had a good record of attending the antenatal clinic at Homa Bay District Hospital but the treatment did not provide a cure. Upon this, her parents referred her to this TBA whom Mary promptly started consulting. The TBA remained "my doctor during the rest of the pregnancy period", she intimated. Mary took herbal medicine and the abdominal pains subsided.

---

*Some names of people and places in this section have been disguised to protect the confidentiality of the informants.

However, she did not stop going to the antenatal clinic, – her last attendance was on September 14, 1989 barely three days before delivery. Nonetheless, it was not her plan to deliver at a hospital maternity ward. "My intention was to deliver here and not at the hospital," she noted and added, "I went to the hospital but they did not give me proper treatment which could cure my pains." However, she confessed that she likes the hospital but "the way they treat people sometimes is not good."

The TBA, who was then seeing eight women daily, had a long-standing reputation in the community as a helper. This attracted Mary's parents and the other women who consulted her for massaging, palpating, medicine and normal pregnancy check-up. Mary's quick and problem-free delivery was facilitated by the TBA's herbal medicine. This was given during labour, not to reduce pain but to hasten delivery. At the time of the interview, she was preparing to go home after a day or two and would take the child to a biomedical facility for postnatal health care.

Case 2: Teresa

Teresa, 24 years old, married with two children, educated up to Standard seven (in the previous education school system) and a follower of the Pentecostal Assemblies of God Church was another interviewee. She came from Kayambo-Kwamo Sub-location, Kanyamwa-Kosewe Location in Ndhiwa Division. She was admitted at the Ralang Village, home of traditional healer Owino, on July 23, 1989, suffering from headache and mental illness. During my interview with her on September 20, 1989, she said that she had been taken there by her brother-in-law.

Teresa's first bout of the same illness occurred in 1986 whereby she experienced severe headache and fever. She went for treatment at Ndhiwa Health Centre and recovered. When she got ill again in 1989, she did not go to a biomedical facility but her brother-in-law took her for prayers at Kirubi Church. Teresa confessed that she was beaten at the church, presumably to exorcise evil spirits. The day after the church experience, she was taken to the home of the traditional healer. At the time of "admission" she was a very violent patient and was chained for a period of two and a half weeks on starting to receive treatment.

Asked why she did not go to a biomedical facility, Teresa said that her brother-in-law "refused and brought me here", "I don't know why he refused to take me to the hospital". Since her admission into Owino's home, her husband who worked in Nakuru, had come to see her once. It is her mother-in-law who visited her frequently. At the time of the interview, Teresa felt much better and could be discharged. Traditional healer Owino attributed the cause of Teresa's illness to *ndagla*–i.e. bewitching.

Case 3: John

John was from Karungu and had completed Form four in 1987 at Maawa Technical School. He became sick in June, 1988, when his hands became stiff and he could not bend the arms. He confessed however, that he always experienced headache throughout his school career. He performed rather poorly, scoring fourth division in his ordinary level school certificate examination.

When John, 21 years old and married, became sick, the grandfather prayed for him. Then the grandmother brought herbal medicine which he was forced to drink; the rest was used to massage his stiff arm. After repeated applications, John recovered.

Slightly over one year later, John started to experience a bit of a headache. Soon, he became violent, breaking the glass windows of his step mother's house. He remembers that he ran to his uncle's house: " I stoned the door until it broke into pieces". His father took him to Sori Health Centre where he was given an injection. He recalled his utterances to the medical staff: "I told the doctor that he was a black primitive man. "What do you know?" Who is the Prime Minister of Israel?" I asked him.

"The day after that," John continued, "my grandmother said that I should be taken to Miranga to see a traditional healer. I was brought her by my father, mother and step-mother." This is how I caught up with John at the healer's home during my visit there on September 20, 1989, barely four days after his admission. He was chained at the ankle in order to restrain his violence.

John's recent illness history (as noted earlier) had began during June, 1988. He was treated with traditional medicine and obtained a temporary cure. Between September and November, 1988 he was a patient at Mathare Mental Hospital in Nairobi. He had been taken there by his father who was working with a soft drinks manufacturing company. After November, he was attending the clinic as an out-patient while residing at his sister's house in Nairobi. The father returned John to their Karungu home in South Nyanza in January, 1989, where the young man resumed normal rural life of helping in farm chores. He did not get ill again until September, 1989.

In the case of John's illness, the healer assessed that the mental illness was caused by *juogi,* in this case evil spirits of a member of the living dead who had not been appeased, by *jachien* (literally satan), in the form of *ndagla* and/or *nawi.*

Case 4: Melisa

At the time we interviewed Mzee Awiti Owanga on September 21, 1989, at Osodo village, Kabura, bone-setter (*jachomo*) William Oje had been invited to treat him here. Melisa, aged about 32 years, married and without children, had also come as an outpatient to consult the healer. She was a devout Catholic who attended mass regularly, but had not gone to school at all.

Melisa had fallen down and sustained a compound fracture at the ankle on August 4, 1989. She was subsequently carried home from the accident site by her brother-in-law. A local bone-setter Abonyo, was called to her home and massaged her broken ankle with herbal medicines and hot stone wrapped in a towel. This process went on daily for one month. There had been little improvement and the family then decided to take her to another bone-setter, Mrs. Odera, 25 kilometers away. She stayed at Mrs. Odera's home for about 2 weeks within which time she started walking a bit. (She had been unable to walk when she was brought to Odera's home).

In the meantime, Melisa's husband heard about William Oje's superior skills at bone-setting. Consequently he went to Odera's home and retrieved Melisa and took her to Oje. She informed me that she had been taken from Odera's home with bones protruding from the affected ankle. Oje was called to attend to her from September 19, 1989. He set the protruding bones to their normal position and massaged the ankle with herbal medicine. He then bandaged the ankle with a piece of cloth. At the time of the interview, she was feeling better although she still felt pain. Melisa's affected leg was still swollen from the foot to the middle of the leg but she could walk with the help of a stick.

Melisa did not go to the hospital because she had been told that traditional bone setters doid a better job. However the decision to seek therapy was made by her brother-in-law, a decision which the husband did not oppose.
Melisa had in the past been admitted to Nyanza Provincial Hospital in Kisumu suffering from abdominal pains but could not remember the dates. However, she recalled that her husband had taken her there. They did not try traditional healers for that illness and she had gotten well.

Melisa thought that the current fracture was just an accident. So far; "I am very happy with the treatment given by my current doctor," she said, beaming with happiness as she visibly suppressed the pain from the ankle.

Case 5: Brenda

Brenda, a nursery school going child and second born of a young couple, fell down on July 5, 1989, while playing with other children and sustained a fracture at the elbow joint. She was promptly rushed to Homa Bay District Hospital, where her arm was plastered and she was returned home. Five weeks later, she was taken back to the hospital where the plaster was removed.

Brenda was born on November 4, 1984. At the time of the interview she was accompanied by her parents. Her father aged 28 years, was a clerk at the Ndhiwa government office. Her mother, 26 years old, belonged to the Seventh Day Adventist Church and had accompanied Brenda for therapy with *jachomo* William Oje. Both parents came from the neighbouring district.

According to her mother, (who narrated the case history and answered my questions), X-ray pictures had shown that Brenda's elbow bones had been severed. After the removal of the plaster, the arm was loose and twisted. She noted that: "the doctor advised us not to worry as physical exercises would eventually make the arm return to its position."

While crediting the hospital treatment for reducing the initial swelling of the arm and confirming that it was already broken, Brenda's parents "did not trust the doctor's advice" that the arm would return to normal with time. Consequently, they were unanimous in the decision to consult a traditional bone-setter. Shortly after the plaster had been removed from Brenda's arm, the parents proceeded to a vacation at their ancestral Kano home in Kisumu. This is where they consulted bone-setter, Awinja. He twisted Brenda's arm to position and held the elbow with a set of sticks tied together (*osembo*) which healers use instead of the hospital plaster. Awinja then put Brenda on a course of daily physiotherapy for two weeks.

When the father's leave elapsed, the family abandoned therapy and returned to Ndhiwa. They began to look for another bone-setter. The mother contended that Brenda's bones had not returned to position during Awinja's therapy. This is how they discovered William Oje.

Table 6.2 provides a summary of the basic characteristics of clients of traditional medicine. This summary comprising 26 people includes the five case histories discussed above.

Table 6.2: Basic characteristics of consumers of traditional medicine in South Nyanza

Patient	Sex	Age	Educational Background: Literate	Educational Background: Illiterate*	1st choice of Therapy: TM	1st choice of Therapy: MM	Therapy Manager Family/Relative	Complaint	Distance to the Healer (Km)
1. Lina	F	18	X			X	X	Evil spirits (Satan)	–
2. Ann	F	18		X		X	X	Chronic gonorrhoea	–
3. Maria	F	35			X		X	Mental illness	–
4. Jimmy	M	24	X			X	X	Mental Illness	–
5. Judy	F	24	X			X	X	Mental Illness	–
6. Anyango	F	48			X		X	Fracture of ankle	–
7. Victor	M	16	X		X		X	Mental Illness	
8. Mary	F	20	X		X		X	Antenatal care; delivery	25
9. Teresa	F	24	X	X			X	Severe headache; mental illness	6
10. John	M	21	X		X		X	Severe headache; mental illness	26
11. Melisa	F	32		X	X		X	Compound fracture	–
12. Brenda	F	5	X**		X		X	Arm fracture	3
13. Owanga	M	57	X		X		Self	Spinal injury; stroke	Called the healer to his home
14. Jane	F	28		X			X	Abdominal pain	40
15. Mercy	F	25	X	X			X	Lower abdominal pain	3
16. Nancy	F	19	X	X		X		Abdominal pain	3
17. Carol	F	25	X			X	X	Joint pains	
18. Nelly	F	20	X			X	X	Abdominal pain, backache	31/2

Patient	Sex	Age	Educational Background Literate	 Illiterate*	1st choice of Therapy TM	 MM	Therapy Manager Family/Relative	Complaint	Distance to the Healer (Km)
19. Lisa	F	25	X			X	Self	Failureto get pregnant; abdominal pain infertility	25
20. Irene	F	15		X	X		Self	Skin rashes all over the body	6
21. Mary-Ann	F	49		X		X	X	Lower abdominal pain and backache	1
22. Tabitha	F	18		X	X		X	Boils all over the body	1
23. Roselyn	F	55		X	X		X	Peptic ulcer	1/2
24. Janet	F	40				X	X	Abortion	0.5
25. Emily	F	30	X		X		Self	Headache; dizziness; tiredness	10
26. Petronilla	F	N/A		X	X		Self	Boils on both feet and legs	5

KEY

* Any person with at least primary education (seven years) is considered literate

** Parents were literate

MM modern medicine

TM traditional medicine

SOURCE: Own field data

Observations

From the foregoing, it is apparent that both literate and illiterate members of the community seek traditional medicine. With regard to the illness that took these patients to the traditional healer, the first choice of therapy was modern medicine rather than traditional medicine. Thus, the latter system is relegated to the second level (i.e. the second level of resort) for most patients. However, it is worth noting that some of the patients expect instantaneous, almost mechanical recovery; they do not seem to wait long enough to complete a course of therapy in a health facility before taking the same episode of illness to traditional medicine. Also, many patients do not stop using drugs from health facilities as they begin to use the herbal medicines. These can be dangerous to the patients concerned because they may cause overdosing by potent mixtures.

It is significant to note that most of the complaints taken to traditional healers are related to mental illness, infertility and abdominal pains. The bulk of female patients suffer from infertility and abdominal pains while mental illness is shared between the sexes.

In almost all the cases, the decision to seek therapy in traditional medicine was made by self and/or a family member (husband, wife, sister, brother etc.) and not a friend.

Turning specifically to the five case histories discussed above, it appears that therapy-seeking behaviour is quite fluid. For example, Mary is a well-educated woman by virtue of her high school education. As an expectant mother, she goes to the antenatal clinic regularly. When she develops abdominal pains, she tries the hospital but does not obtain a cure and resorts to traditional medicine and succeeds. However, she does not stop attending the antenatal clinic and instead she moves freely between traditional medicine and the hospital. Also she will take her child to a postnatal health clinic. Her case demonstrates the way patients use various medical systems in a complementary way. She sticks to the hospital for antenatal and postnatal care for her child. However, she seeks traditional medicine as it is efficacious for her abdominal problem and besides she likes the personal attention that she receives from the healer.

The problem of abdominal pains during pregnancy *(tuo ich)* is among the conditions which the Luo believe cannot be cured by modern medicine. The other diseases in this category are mental illness (*neko*), abdominal pains caused by evil eye (*ich muor*), epilepsy *(ndulume)*, postpartum abdominal pains (*ojiwo*), and women infertility (*dhako maok nyuol*). Mary's therapy manager (her own mother) obviously is aware of this and directs the patients to a reputable healer.

Teresa's case history again shows how patients first seek therapy in biomedicine and move on to traditional medicine during another episode of the same illness. Teresa went to hospital, then to church (for prayers), and finally to a traditional healer. It is significant to note, as Janzen (1978) found among the Bakongo of lower Zaire, that the decision to seek therapy, and where to seek it, does not lie with the patient, but is made by the lay therapy-managing group comprising family members and/or close friends. In Teresa's case, therapy was managed by her elder brother-in-law and apparently the mother-in-law. The husband, then working some 300 kilometers (in Nakuru) was only told of the progress of his wife's illness.

John's case is somewhat similar to that of Teresa. He is taken ill, his grandmother administers traditional medicine and in the subsequent episode of the illness, his father seeks therapy at a health centre. Thereafter, the grandmother insists that he be taken to a specific healer. Apparently, in both cases of Teresa and John, it is the other family members who appear to be influential in selecting therapy for the patient.

The case of Melisa is somewhat different from the others in the sense that her injury is physical. Melisa's brother-in-law takes her to a bone-setter. After observing little improvement, the husband retrieves her and takes her to another bone-setter who is thought to be more skilled. The therapy managers in this case have not thought about biomedicine, perhaps because they take traditional therapy to be more efficacious for fractures especially those involving adults.

On the other hand, Brenda's case demonstrates the winding course of therapy – from hospital to traditional healer and to another traditional healer. The parents become dissatisfied with hospital therapy as the child's arm bones do not appear to have gone back to normal position. Sceptical about biomedical advice and anxious to obtain full recovery for their child as early as possible, the parents seek therapy in another realm. Brenda's parents could not wait lest the problem persisted and she became an adult with a twisted arm. Her parents, however, give credit to biomedicine for reducing the swelling on the arm and diagnosing accurately that her bones were separated.

Conclusion

This inquiry into why the Luo go to traditional healers shows that therapy-seeking and therapy-selecting behaviour is quite pragmatic. The disease aetiologies discussed earlier provide pointers to conceptualizing and gaining deeper insights into disease and illness categories as conceived within a culture. The classification itself is theoretical and intuitive (see Chapter 2 and 3). When faced with actual sickness, the Luo tend to try whatever therapies promise relief and the restoration of health.

Culture is in transition as the forces of Western education, Christianity and contact with the outside world exert their influence on the society. These have modified the observance or otherwise of certain customs, traditions and taboos through altering values and terms of reference. Ultimately, these processes affect therapy-seeking behaviour.

In the wake of these societal changes, there have also been a number of transitional diseases and illnesses; some hitherto were unknown to the community, whereas symptoms may be difficult to distinguish one from another. This creates the need for a pragmatic search through the available therapies to restore health.

Tradition persists among the educated. There is also the situation commonly encountered where parents are illiterate and the offspring are well educated. The older people hold strong beliefs that certain diseases cannot be cured in biomedicine and hence they will seek treatment in traditional medicine for their educated kin.

Also, the course of therapy-seeking is not always systematic; frequently, all the available medical systems are utilized simultaneously for the same episode of illness.

The findings of this inquiry have important implications to health care planning; planning should take into account the fact that people tend to utilize most of the health resources available in a community. For example, if expectant mothers feel more comfortable with traditional birth attendants, the latter's vocation should be studied, enhanced and made safer rather than replacing it wholesale. The same can be said of traditional bone-setters (or physiotherapists) and herbalists.

The findings have also showed that the majority of the people first resort to modern medicine before consulting traditional healers. Assuming that biomedical workers can provide expected care and adopt a more personal and warm approach to patients, it would appear that the numbers going to traditional medicine before the initial course of therapy is complete would be reduced. The biomedical staff must however, be ready to explain the time lag between the time the treatment process commences and the expected time of recovery. Many patients and their families tend to be impatient; they expect instantaneous recovery.

REFERENCES

Ampofo, O. and F. D. Johnson-Romauld. 1978. *Traditional Medicine and Its Role in the Development of Health Services in Africa*. Background paper for the Technical Discussion of the 25th, 26th and the 27th Sessions of the Regional Committee for Africa. Brazzaville: World Health Organization Regional Office for Africa.

Fabrega, H. 1982. "A Commentary on African System of Medicine." In *African Health and Healing Systems* Edited by P. S. Yoder. Los Angeles: Crossroads Press. pp. 237-252.

Foster, M. 1976. "Disease Aetiologies in Non-Western Medical Systems" *American Anthropologist* 78 No. 4: 773-782.

Janzen, M. 1978. *The Quest for Therapy: Medical Pluralism in Lower Zaire*. Berkeley: University of California Press.

Kenya, Government of. 1989. *South Nyanza Development Plan 1989-1993*. Nairobi: Ministry of Planning and National Development.

___________.n.d. 1979. *Population Census Vol. 11: Analytical Report*. Nairobi: Central Bureau of Statistics.

K'okul, R. N. O. 1991. *Maternal and Child Health in Kenya: A Study of Poverty, Disease and Malnutrition in Samia*. Helsinki: The Finnish Society for Development Studies and Scandinavian Institute of African Studies.

Mbiti, J. S. 1969. *African Religions and Philosophy*. London: Heinemann.

Ocholla-Ayayo, A. B. C. 1976. *Traditional Ideology and Ethics Among the Southern Luo*. Uppsala: Scandinavian Institute of African Studies.

Odada, J. E. and J. O. Otieno (eds). 1990. *Socio-Economic Profiles*. Nairobi: Ministry of Planning and National Development and UNICEF (Kenya Country Office.)

Sindiga, I. 1985. "The Persistence of High Fertility in Kenya" *Social Science and Medicine* 20 No. 1:71-84.

______. 1992. *Ethnomedicine and Health Care in Kenya*. Final Technical Report to the International Development Research Centre for project No. 3-P-87-0231. Eldoret: Moi University.

Whisson, M. G. 1974. "Some Aspects of Functional Disorders Among the Kenya Luo." *In Magic, Faith and Healing: Studies in Primitive Psychiatry Today* edited by A. Kiev. New York: Free Press. pp. 293-304.

Yoder, P. 1982. "Issues in the Study of Ethnomedical Systems in Africa". In *African Health and Healing Systems* edited by P. S. Yoder. Los Angeles: Crossroads Press. pp. 1-20.

Chapter 7

ETHNOMEDICAL REMEDIES AND THERAPIES IN MATERNAL AND CHILD HEALTH AMONG THE RURAL LUO*

Evelynes Agot Kawango

The purpose of this chapter is to investigate how the rural community participates in its health care by using indigenous medical resources with regard to mothers and children. The chapter identifies the common maternal and childhood health problems experienced, their perceived causes and the remedies sought.

Health and Disease Among the Luo

The concept of health encompasses all aspects that contribute to preventive and curative care. Health is not the mere absence of disease or infirmity, but a state of complete physical, mental and social well-being; it is a dynamic quality continually changing to cope with and adapt to social and physical environments (Meade et. al., 1989:8-9).

The quest for this mental, physical and social well-being is inherent in man and this implies that human quest for therapy is more ancient than formal institutional health facilities. Through time, each culture has developed mechanisms of coping with disease and illness. The Luo have preventive, adaptive and curative strategies to cope with ill-health, drawing from their culture and the ecological environment. To them, people's behaviour and interpersonal relationships are directly linked with their health status. They have regulations

* I am greatly indebted to my 44 informants, particularly the childless, who kindly shared with me, in word, their personal trauma and to Mzee Japolo the diviner who let me observe him at work. Special thanks also to Dr. Edwin Were, Alex Amolo and Anastasia Auma for further editing and demonstration. And to Kimuma, for speedy typing.

governing all aspects of behaviour including married life, pregnancy and sexual relations. Any violations of the above have specific health implications demanding certain remedies and therapies.

Ethnomedical remedies and therapies are varied and all-encompassing; there is no aspect of life that exists independent of health. The guiding feature of behaviour is (*kwer* pl. *kweche*), meaning a forbidden act or taboo. There is always caution as to whether what one does or is expected to do is *kwer* or not.

Following Sindiga's taxonomy of disease aetiologies among the Luo (see Chapter 6), I will specify which diseases in each category affect mothers and children. This is a prelude to the discussion on medicine with regard to maternal child health.

Methods

I carried out a small survey in September and October, 1992, to gain information on the use of traditional therapies. I selected 38 women of childbearing age 16 of whom had lost at least one child below age five, 19 had children below age 5, and 3 were childless. Three traditional birth attendants, two female herbalists and one male diviner were also interviewed. The interviews were done in Bar-Chando, Abom and Ajigo Sub-locations in North Sakwa Location, and Usigu Sub-location in Central Yimbo Location Bondo Division, Siaya District.

The questions elicited information on the socio-economic background of the respondents; where they delivered each child and why they chose the place/facility; common children's diseases and their causes; where they sought therapy and reasons behind their choice; whether they have changed therapy; traditional therapy sought and fees paid. Those who had lost a child were asked what caused the death and the treatment the child received before death. The mothers were also asked whether they had problems with conception, the cause and remedy sought. Questions for the traditional birth attendants and the diviner dealt with their specializations, where their clients came from, what maternal and childhood health problems they handled, and what they charged for the services.

Findings

Based on the above survey, this section discusses common health problems among mothers and children, their perceived causes and subsequent management.

Common maternal health problems and remedies

Infertility or sub-fertility is the most serious maternal problem. Mbiti (1969:133-4) observes that for African people, marriage is the focus of existence, and that marriage and procreation are a unity; without procreation, marriage is incomplete. It follows that inability to bear children is the greatest misfortune among women.

Sindiga's (1992) classification of disease aetiologies entirely apply in the understanding of causes of infertility or sub-fertility (see also chapter 6). The infertility problem may result from human causes (i.e. *Lwet dhano*). Destructive charms may be obtained from *jandagla* or *janawi* to 'tie' (*tweyo/tudo*) the womb of somebody. The concept of *tudo*, however, does not apply to infertility alone. One may 'tie' somebody so that he/she does not marry, go to school, pass examinations, secure a job and so on. In these cases, any item which has been in physical contact with the victim's body such as a piece of cloth, shoes, soil from foot-marks (*lop tielo*), pen or book or part of the body such as nails, hair (especially pubic hair), urine and stool, are discretely obtained for use by the sorcerers in causing the infertility.

Infertility may also be caused by the spirits of the living dead (*juogi*) whereby the ancestral spirits may refuse to "open the womb" of a woman if they have been offended by either of the couple and/or their relative(s). For instance, if a son/daughter marries from/into a sworn enemy's family, the spirits might be angered and revenge by making the couple childless. In other words, the ancestors would not want to be perpetuated from such a union. If the parents or grandparents of the childless couple were witches (*jojuogi*) or sorcerers (*jondagla/janawi*), this could be a punishment meted out by the victims who died from their witchcraft. (They always say that *joma otho ok nindi/joma otho neno*— the dead are not asleep/the dead do see.)

Another cause of infertility may be breaching of taboos and customs. This takes many forms; for example, marrying a blood relative, however far the link is. Traditionally, relationships were traced back to the founders of clans and all descendants were related to each other, as a mother or a father, sister or bother, aunt or uncle, grandmother or grandfather. Marriage was not even allowed between members of different clans whose founders were brothers or cousins. *Ok wakendre/nyuomore gi jo dhood x* (we do not marry from/into clan x) is used to designate continuing blood relationship (*wat*) among/between certain clans as this would be tantamount to incest. Ocholla-Ayayo (1976:104) says that incest is one of the highest order of offences in the society, resulting in *chira* (see Sindiga elsewhere in this volume) which may prevent a woman from giving birth at all, or cause a miscarriage, still-birth or lead to death of infants. If fertility does arise in such a union, children born may be physically and/or mentally handicapped.

Sub-fertility may occur if the wife has a child outside the marriage bond. The Luo have a ritual called *kalo nyathi* where the parents place the child between them on their bed sometime after delivery so that if it was conceived on another bed (implying conception by another man), then either the baby would die from *chira* or the mother would stop having more children or both. This belief helped to check unfaithfulness in women.

Also, infertility may be genetically perpetuated. Childless female relatives of a wife were seen as signs that the problem was somewhere in the blood and this was and still is known to have ended marriage negotiations. Acute menstrual pain, *segete*, is also believed to delay the first conception, while abdominal ailments from *yamo* (literally, boils associated with wind and seasonal changes) usually cause sub-fertility but may also lead to complete infertility. However, malnutrition, as a cause of infertility (Sindiga, 1985; Golapan and Rao, 1985) has hardly been conceptualized by the rural Luo.

From the discussion on the causes of infertility, it is apparent that besides inherited and *yamo*-related infertility, the other causes are human induced, either through a curse, an envious person or from the victim's action (or inaction) and/or that of her husband or their relatives. Spring (1980), Good (1980; 1987) and Sindiga (1992) have reported that diseases of human origin are believed to be best managed by traditional medicine. Thus herbal medicine is the first line of therapy taken to remove the impurities from the womb and cure the *yamo*. If the condition persists, other causes are suspected, in which case a diviner (*jakoro*) is consulted to decipher the cause. He uses cowrie shells (*gagi*) and other paraphernalia, plus a gourd (*puga*) where the spirits (*juogi*) "reside" and are invoked to reveal the cause(s). These may fall within human agency, ancestral spirits or from breaching of taboos and customs. Once the cause is revealed, the diviner prescribes the most suitable therapy or refers the individual to a traditional healer (*ajuoga*).

Causes through human intervention call for the destruction of the spell. This therapy involves the ritual of untying (*gonyo*) of the charm that tied the womb through sacrifices and other ritual manipulations, accompanied by herbal medicines and sometimes ash (*buru*) from some concoction with the power to ward off evil. At times, this operation involves the counter-tying (*loko*) of the sorcerer and his client who caused the spell so that they do not re-tie the now-released woman. This vicious cycle of tying, untying, re-tying and counter-tying may continue until a weaker, less patient party gives up.

If the diviner diagnosed the source of the problem to be the living dead, the curse is usually removed by acts of appeasement by cleansing to placate the spirits (*juogi*) for the offence committed or by a ritual of scattering of the spell (*loko dhoch*). If the cause involves disregarding a taboo (*kwer*), this must cease for the therapy to be effective. A concoction of special, powerful herbs (*manyasi*) is given to dispel the 'crime' caused by the breach of the taboo. This is called *hoso*. *Manyasi* is therefore not meant to identify the underlying cause of a disease

(Sindiga, 1992:245), but to cure an already identified cause or to abort an impending health consequence, *chira*. Note that only minor *chira (chira matindo)* can be cured or aborted but major *chira (chira maduong/madongo)* has no remedy (Sindiga, 1992; Ocholla-Ayayo, 1976).

The struggle by a childless woman can be exasperating. All possible remedies are explored and exploited until there is no hope. Mbiti (1969:110-11) notes that unhappy is a woman who fails to get children, for whatever qualities she might possess, this failure to bear children renders her a dead end of a human life on both the genealogical line and her own line since nobody from her blood will remember her and keep her in a constant state of personal immortality when she dies (*kare otho nono*). Mbiti adds that childlessness is an irreparable humiliation for which there is no source of comfort in traditional life, and even if it is the husband at fault, the wife is not excused in the eyes of the society.

During pregnancy, the woman must observe certain taboos and regulations to protect herself and the unborn child. One of the leading regulations relates to sexual relationships, for example, the assertion that sex outside wedlock may lead to miscarriage (*ich wuok*) or ante-partum haemorrhage (*ich ma chwer*—the womb which is leaking) in which case *manyasi* and other herbs are administered.

These two problems mentioned above may also be caused in the same way as infertility, and hence therapy seeking would be similar. Also, protective charm (*bilo*) may be worn or rubbed into small cuts on the skin (*saro*) to ward off any harmful intent by man or evil spirits (*jochiende*) towards the mother and the unborn child. Abdominal problems may also lead to miscarriages and these are believed to be best treated by traditional birth attendants, *(nyamrerwa*). It should be noted that the TBAs have multiple roles: traditional midwives, obstetricians, gynaecologists and paediatricians. Although most popularly used in reference to a TBA, the term *nyamrerwa* is also used in the context of a personal doctor and counsellor on general health matters.

Another stage where traditional therapeutics come in handy is during birth. Choosing TBAs to manage pregnancy and/or birth continues to be significant in many African countries (Good, 1980a; 1987; Sindiga, 1992). Several reasons are cited for opting for traditional midwives; of the 35 mothers with whom I had in-depth discussions, 11 (31.4%) preferred TBAs although nearly all of them attended both antenatal and postnatal clinics. Three (8.6%) delivered on their own, assisted by relatives and neighbours but they too admitted having attended both ante and postnatal clinics. The remaining 21 (60%) delivered in health centres. Of the latter, 18 (88.9%) had used herbs at one stage or other for pregnancy-related problems and thus the implication is clear; both biomedical and ethnomedical therapies are used for the same episode of illness either in sequence or in parallel. Similar findings are reported by Spring (1980), Good (1980; 1987) and Sindiga (1992).

Reasons given by those who used TBAs ranged from consideration of distance and cost, unavailability of drugs and indifference of the medical staff. Most TBAs give herbal medicine to lessen labour pains (*yadh muoch*) and hasten birth, an element they claim lacks altogether in modern health institutions. TBAs are also good in difficult births without being 'theatre-eager' (i.e. running for the knife to perform cesarean sections as is common in maternity hospitals). When the baby lies in a wrong position, either squatting (*gumo*) or feet first (*dhoch*), these midwives are adept at identifying and correcting the anomaly during antenatal visits or during birth. It is only when delivery is exceptionally difficult or when serious complications arise after delivery that hospitals may be helpful. However, this may be too late.

Moreover, TBAs are preferred because they give herbal medicine to expel retained placenta, to reduce post-partum abdominal pains (*ojiwo*), and to aid breast-milk production. These experts are also prompt in disentangling the umbilical cord (*wino*) from the neck of the baby so that blood flow is not interfered with during birth. In short, TBAs are preferred over hospital-trained midwives not only because of their accessibility, affordability and good personal relations, but also because of their apparently sound knowledge in maternal child health care.

One of the major criticisms against TBAs is their low level of hygiene. However, the Government of Kenya and various non-governmental organizations (NGOs), notably AMREF and UNICEF, are conducting training programmes for them. But the training programmes which take the seminar or workshop approach, have been criticized by old practitioners, who argue that their school-like nature befits only their younger, literate counterparts. They suggest that since they (the older practitioners) are very few, they would benefit more by visits in their homes by trainers, although they are sceptical as to whether there is anything new they still need to learn.

The inability of TBAs to control internal haemorahage, a factor that has been cited as the greatest cause of maternal deaths, particularly in the prenatal and postnatal periods (UNEP, 1991:235), militates against them as well. Neonatal tetanus from open wounds is the second leading cause of death among the vaccine-preventable diseases (UNEP, 1991-237), and yet the TBAs apply soot *(oyare)*, ember (*mirni*) or herbs to cover and protect the navel wound (umbilical stump). Eye infections at birth from infected birth canal is treated by smoke from smoldering medicinal plants directed at the eye.

Common childhood health problems and remedies

Infant and childhood diseases may be classified into four major categories on the basis of their perceived sources and specialised therapies required in their management. These are (i) environmental diseases which include infectious and respiratory diseases; (ii) metabolic and nutritional disorders; (iii) diseases requiring surgical manipulations; and (iv) miscellaneous diseases from an array of factors, such as inheritance, human agencies, ancestral spirits and breaching taboos.

Environmental diseases

Infectious diseases of parasitic nature include malaria *(del maowore/ma chwakore* in reference to increase in body temperature) and other feverish conditions *(midhusu)*, stomachache *(ichkach/muor)*, amoebiasis, intestinal candidiasis *(mgongo)*, diarrhoea *(diep)*, thrush *(orianyancha)*, roundworms *(njokni/njohni)*, ringworms *(odhuedho)*, scabies *(guonyo)* and dysentery *(ndira)*. All the 35 mothers interviewed cited malaria, always present in half the children in Nyanza (Kenya, 1989:66), as being best treated by biomedical remedies, usually self-prescribed shop drugs. There are also traditional herbs that treat malaria; the leaves, bark and roots are boiled and part of the solution taken orally while the other is used to steam the patient, to 'sweat out the fever', so to speak. The process is called *fundo/humo*.

Diarrhoea is not a disease *per-se* but a symptom of a problem in the gastro-intestinal tract (Thompson, 1968; K'Okul, 1991). Nevertheless, it is a cause to 28% (or 4 million) deaths in children annually world-wide (UNEP, 1991:238). Diarrhoea may result from many diseases, the common ones being thrush *(orianyacha)*, amoebiasis and other parasitic infections, all of which are believed to come from the use of and contact with polluted water as well as from eating soil. Seventy seven per cent (N = 35) of the mothers reported diarrhoeal diseases as being common among their children, confirming the findings of the national health survey of 1989 (Kenya, 1989:64) which ranked Nyanza Province second to Western in the occurrence of diarrhoea. Herbal therapy is recommended, not simply for stopping diarrhoea, but also for treating the underlying cause; for example, in thrush, the faeces would be slimy, some of the roundworms may be vomited and/or excreted. In amoebiasis, the faeces is usually frothy and may be laced with blood while in intestinal candidiasis (*mgongo*) a condition known as prolapse where rectum protrudes may be observed (Thompson, 1968:746). The rectum is made to shrink back into position by splashing or sponging with cold water. Treatment involves boiling herbal medicine (*yadh agulu/achwaka*) and crushing the herbs (*yadh asuaga*) and mixing with water (*yadh abuda*). Some of the solution is taken orally while the rest is put in a basin and the child placed inside. The water near the anus is blown using reeds (*odundu*), with one end immersed in water till it froths. This treatment, called *kudho*, is meant to kill the threadworm which causes anal itching.

Infectious and respiratory diseases are the greatest cause of morbidity and mortality. Globally, they account for over one third of all the deaths, with children under five being the most susceptible (UNEP, 1991:238). Among the contagious diseases, five are common; colds (*athung'a*), coughs (*ahonda*), scabies (*guonyo*), ringworms (*odhuedho/siling*) and measles (*anyiewu/-ang'iewu*). Common colds and slight coughs are often left to disappear on their own. If they persist, herbs or over-the-counter shop drugs are used. For a stubborn cold, medicinal leaves are dried and crushed into powder. Dosage of small pinches are put into the nostrils or the powder is made into a solution and dropped into the nostrils *(fito/biyo/bicho)*. The severe sneezing that follows is expected to stop the runny nose and clear the cold by killing the worms (*kute*) in the head that bring the problems (see also discussion on *sambwa* below). Both ringworms and scabies are treated by applying herbal medicines, crushed and mixed with petroleum jelly (for adhesiveness) to the affected area. Some of the herbs are taken orally in solution.

The biggest terror of the contagious diseases is measles. It is believed that if measles is not treated fully, it remains chronic and may later cause blindness. Thirty one mothers (N=35) felt that measles can only be treated by traditional herbs, and that modern medicine hastens death rather than recovery! They claimed that hospital staff often read the wrong symptoms and give 'some injections which makes the disease hide in the stomach' (*ma pando tuo e ich*), killing the child shortly afterwards. They recommended herbal drinks to speed up the clinical skin symptoms so that it may be treated effectively. Of the 16 mothers who had lost at least one child before the age of five, 11 (68.8%) quoted measles as the cause of the deaths. Seven of these (63.6%) had been taken to hospital, mistaking the symptoms for malaria. Three of the remaining four did not identify the disease in time and relied on self prescribed shop drugs and one started using the herbs too late.

In both parasitic and contagious diseases, environmental sanitation is a key determinant and yet Nyanza Province leads in obtaining water from unprotected sources, ranks second to Coast Province in poor housing conditions, and ranks third in having no toilet facilities (Kenya, 1989; 71; 1992:182). K'Okul (1991: 39) found that diarrhoea in Samia occurred because mothers drank and cooked with water contaminated with faecal coliform and other pollutants. This was the underlying cause of infections such as amoebiasis and cholera. Respiratory diseases, mainly pneumonia, are identified by difficulty in breathing (*thung'*) and coughing. Nyanza Province ranks second after Rift Valley in the frequency of respiratory diseases (Kenya, 1989:69).

In cases of respiratory diseases, biomedical services are prefered in acute cases (see also Springs, 1980) and over-the-counter shop drugs and/or herbs are used in cases of mild chest infections. Serious coughs – tuberculosis (*kahera*), and whooping cough (*ahonda guogi*, the cough of the dogs, perhaps a reference to the barking sound made) may be taken to health centres if the two lines of therapy fail.

Most parasitic and contagious (including some respiratory) problems which cause high morbidity and mortality are actually vaccine preventable. The WHO Expanded Programme in Immunization (EPI), which was adopted in Kenya in 1981, is an essential part of child health care. Despite this campaign, Nyanza Province has a poor record of full immunization (Kenya, 1989:64).

Metabolic and nutritional disorders

Metabolic and nutritional disorders are; *mbaha/woyo* (mild to moderate malnutrition), *akuodi/hudha* (acute malnutrition), *hima* (enlarged spleen from chronic malaria and/or schistosomiasis) a continuous painful and *mbunda*, and dilated belly, both in pregnant women and children, caused by frequent indigestion and accumulation of gas), *hero* (general weakness of a child following close birth interval) and *remo ma rumo* (anemia). In the mother, these disorders may lead to underweight babies of less than 2.5 kilogrammes, a condition which leads to higher mortality compared with heavier babies in the first year of life (UNEP, 1991:236). In fact, none of the mothers interviewed ever had any special diet during pregnancy.

Apart from anaemic conditions which are understood to be caused by little and/or poor quality food and constipation which is easily relieved by herbal medicine, the other nutritional disorders are interpreted as *yamo*.

Hero is the weakening of a child whose mother becomes pregnant soon after its birth. The length of birth intervals has a strong effect on infant and childhood morbidity and mortality levels. *Chuny mopodho* (the liver has collapsed) is a conceived health episode. This 'disease' is associated with thin, *weakly-looking* people, with hollow epigastrium. Such people, it is maintained, cannot become healthy unless the "collapsed liver" has been 'erected' by an expert. The traditional healer would ritually hoist the liver (*pidho/chungo chuny mopodho*). A bean or greengram seed is then planted beneath a pot of drinking water or near a banana plant. Once the seed germinates, it symbolically implies that the 'collapsed liver' has also germinated and the child or adult begins to recover.

Incidentally, these health problems are believed to be caused by *yamo* or in rare cases, inherited as a punishment from the parents who were sorcerers. Due to *yamo*, and possibly the ancestral spirits, traditional therapies take precedence over the modern ones.

Surgical cases

Childhood diseases requiring surgical manipulations include those which need removal or excision, such as uvula (*lim*), extra digit(s) (*katunga/ndunga*) and milk teeth which come too early (*jimo*), and those which need incision such as boils (*buche*), removal of burrowed and worms cutaneous myosis (*kute*), removal of toxic food from the stomach of a bewitched person (*tako*) and small cuts on the skin (*saro*) to rub on protective or curative charm.

When the milk teeth appear too early, they make the child develop acute diarrhoea and vomiting. Hospital syrups are not absorbed and are vomited or get out through diarrhoea. The baby gets heavily dehydrated, does not eat and wastes away fast. Because the medication is neither absorbed nor digested, biomedical remedies are believed to be ineffective and it is claimed that hospital staff are not able to diagnose the illness at all. When it is detected early, it can be retarded (*thiro*) by pressing the gum with herbal medicines. When the teeth have come out, they must be extracted (*nak/nago*) by a special traditional surgeon called *janak*.

An extra digit or stump (*sundo*) should be cut off immediately after birth so that the pain is minimized. Herbs with antiseptic properties are applied on the wound to keep it germ-free and hasten the healing process. Boils are made to ripen quickly when covered with cobweb, after which they are cut open (*baro*) and pus drained out. Cutaneous myosis (or burrowed worms) are usually contracted from urine-soaked mats or earthen floors where children sleep. The skin where they have burrowed is slit open and the worm removed. The small skin perforation is left to heal by itself. Inflamed uvula causes an irritative cough, itching and frequent sore throat. It is tied with hair from a cow's tail (*wino mar iw dhiang'*) and severed with a razor blade fixed at one end of a stick.

The Luo believe that there are people, usually women, with evil eyes (*juog wang'/sihoho*) who possess the power to bewitch the food somebody is eating so that it becomes toxic in the stomach. Thus, this disease conception is culture-specific. The 'infected' child develops severe stomachache and constipation. There are three indigenous solutions to this: One, somebody with suitable herbs neutralizes the toxic effects (*hoso*). Two, if the *jasihoho* is known, she may be brought and forced to talk to the child or give *anti-sihoho* herbs. In both actions the toxin is rendered harmless. The third and more serious situation is the case where the *jasihoho* is not known and a special traditional surgeon known as *jatak* is called to remove the toxic food. He does this by making a small cut near the stomach pit and 'sucks out' the poisonous food either by his mouth or through a horn. How this food is retrieved is a mystery because I observed three children who had the operation and the scars looked superficial. The mothers said the cuts hardly went beyond the skin but that the surgeon did retrieve the food. This is another conceptual and not perceptual health phenomenon. Modern medicine appears powerless in handling this condition. (They say that biomedical personnel do not even know how to diagnose it and these professionals, when faced with *sihoho* cases in their families, often go back to the village to seek ethnomedical therapy).

Miscellaneous diseases

The last category of childhood diseases has varied causes. Health problems from ancestral spirits (*juogi*) include those related to naming *(chako/cheko*) and, at times, convulsions (*sambwa*). When an ancestor wants a child to be named after him/her, the child will cry, refuse food and sleep until this is done. The cause of the restlessness is either revealed in a dream sent by the ancestor in question to one of the relatives or through a diviner.

Sambwa is associated with three causes: One, that necessary herbs were not put in the child's nose (*fito*) early enough to kill the worms believed to be in the head. This is detected when a child sleep-walks, sleep-talks or sleeps fitfully (*buogore ka nindo*). If the worm matures, it leads to convulsions and if left untreated, it may even cause madness (*neko*). Two, displeased ancestors may cause the convulsions as a punishment for some past violations of taboos by the parents or their relatives. It is said that *joma piny/jopiny thage* (the people of the underworld are disturbing him), probably as opposed to *jopolo* (people of the sky/heaven, and therefore of God). Thirdly, a jealous enemy may use witchcraft to cause the disease or re-direct the illness from a suffering member of his family to the new sufferer (*olokne tuo*). If the causes are induced by man (*mag dhano*), by the ancestral spirits (*mag juogi*) or by evil spirits (*mag jo-chiende*) therapy would be similar to those already discussed under infertility. If the cause is natural, treatment is similar to that of a persistent cold but with stronger herbs.

Clinical symptoms of *sambwa* are almost similar to those of epilepsy (*ndulume*) but the latter is believed to be inherited, unless it is redirected as in *sambwa* above.

Okulbat is a state where the baby stretches excessively and frequently, with pain in the joints and the general skeletal structure. If left unattended, the child may later develop a hump and other physical deformities. Herbal medicine (with anti-rheumatic properties) mixed with petroleum jelly is massaged (*rwayo/rwecho*) around the joints. Self-prescribed shop liniments or even soap suds may also be used for the massage.

Conclusion

Among the Luo, most diseases are perceived within the framework of their cultural background. They are explained in terms of human agency through ancestral spirits and from breaching taboos and customs, and not always by Louis Pasteur's germ theory. Biomedical therapy is usually consulted for acute symptoms and natural diseases of inheritance and of the physical environment. Traditional medicine is consulted to deal with underlying causes of human agency, ancestral spirits, evil spirits or breaching taboos. (Similar findings are reported by Rappaport (1980:67). In practice, people make extensive but discriminative use of both therapies concurrently or in sequence (see also Spring, 1980; Good, 1980; 1987; Sindiga, 1992) because symptoms for different diseases overlap and are attributed to different causes depending on the course the illness is taking (cf. Sindiga elsewhere in this volume). The multiple use offers a kind of comprehensive health insurance so that all possible causes are covered simultaneously.

Common maternal health problems treated using traditional medicines and remedies include infertility and sub-fertility and related complications. These may result from breaching taboos, ancestors, anger, the work of witches, infidelity or inheritance. Therapies for these ailments range from herbal medicine to rituals and they aim to undo the harm, appease the ancestors or cleanse a person. Traditional birth attendants (TBAs) are very useful in this field despite the fact that nearly all women attend antenatal and postnatal clinics. Criticism levelled against TBAs in connection with the low level of hygiene does not seem to affect their popularity.

Common childhood problems include environmental diseases such as infectious respiratory disorders, metabolic and nutritional disorders. There are also diseases that require surgical manipulations and diseases from an array of factors such as inheritance, human agencies, ancestral spirits and breaching of taboos. These are treated with herbal medicines and other traditional procedures aimed at correcting the perceived wrong or evil. Surgical manipulations are used to extract digits and constipated food from the stomach as well as milk teeth that appear too early.

The perception of illness by the patients influences the choice of therapy. The have a wide range of therapies to choose from and the choice is made on the basis of the disease and circumstances surrounding its occurrence.

REFERENCES

Cohen, D. W. and E. S. Atieno-Odhiambo. 1989. *Siaya: The Historical Anthropology of an African Landscape*. Nairobi: Heinemann Kenya.

Good, C. M. 1980. "A Comparison of Rural and Urban Ethnomedicine Among the Kamba of Kenya." In *Traditional Health Care Delivery in Contemporary Africa* edited by Priscilla R. Ulin and M. H. Segall. Foreign and Comparative Studies, African Series XXXV. Syracuse: Maxwell School of Citizenship and Public Affairs (Syracuse University).

________________. 1980a. "Ethnomedical Systems in Africa and the LDCs: Key Issues for the Geographer." In *Conception and Methodological Issues in Medical Geography* edited by M.S. Meade. Chapel Hill: University of North Carolina. pp. 93-116.

________________. 1987. *Ethnomedical Systems in Africa: Patterns of Traditional Medicine in Rural and Urban Kenya*. New York: The Guilford Press.

Gopalan, C. and K. J. Rao. 1980. *The Problem of Malnutrition in Childhood in Prevention of Health Problems in Adult Life*. Geneva: WHO.

K'Okul, R. N. O. 1991. *Maternal and Child Health in Kenya – A Study of Poverty, Disease and Malnutrition in Samia*. Helsinki: The Finnish Society for Development Studies and The Scandinavian Institute of African Studies.

Mbiti, J. S. 1969. *African Religions and Philosophy*. London: Heinemann.

Mboya, P. 1938. *Luo Kitgi Gi Timbegi: A Handbook of Luo Customs*. Kisumu: Anyange Press Ltd.

________________. 1978. *Richo Ema Kelo Chira*. Nairobi: East African Publishing House.

Meade, M., J. Florin and W. Gesler. 1988. *Medical Geography*. New York: Guilford Press.

Ogot, G. 1966. *The Promised Land*. Nairobi: East African Publishing House.

Ocholla-Ayayo, A.B.C. 1976. *Traditional Ideology and Ethics Among the Southern Luo*. Uppsala: Scandinavian Institute of African Studies.

Othieno-Ochieng', N.A. 1968. *Luo Social Systems, With a Special Analysis of Marriage Rituals*. Nairobi: Equatorial Publishers Ltd.

Rappaport, H. 1980. "The Integration of Scientific and Traditional Healing: The Problem of De-Mystification." In *Traditional Health Care Delivery in Contemporary Africa* edited by P.R. Ulin and M. H. Segall. Syracuse: Syracuse University. pp. 81-98.

Kenya, Government of. 1992. *Economic Survey, 1992*. Nairobi: Central Bureau of Statistics.

________________. 1989 *Kenya Demographic and Health Survey*. Nairobi: Institute for Resource Development/Micro-systems and National Council for Population and Development and Ministry of Home Affairs and National Heritage.

Sindiga, I. 1992. *Ethnomedicine and Health Care in Kenya*. Final Technical Report to the International Development Research Centres for Project No. 3–P-87-0231. Eldoret: Moi University.

________________. 1985. "The Persistence of High Fertility in Kenya" *Social Science and Medicine* 20, 1: 71-84.

Spring, A. 1980. "Traditional and Biomedical Health Care Systems in Northwest Zambia: A Case of the Luvale." In *Traditional Health Care Delivery in Contemporary Africa* edited by P. R. Ulin and M. H. Segall. Syracuse: Syracuse University. pp. 57-80.

Thompson, W.A.R. 1968. *Black's Medical Dictionary,* 28th Edition. London: Adam and Charles Black.

Ulin, P. R. 1980. "Traditional Healers and Primary Health Care in Africa." In *Traditional Health Care Delivery in Contemporary Africa* edited by P. R. Ulin and M. H. Segall. Syracuse: Syracuse University.

UNEP. 1991. "Human Health". *Environmental Data Report 1991/92*. London: GEMS Monitoring and Assessment Research Centre and World Resource Institute.

Chapter 8

MAASAI TRADITIONAL MEDICINE*

Isaac Sindiga

Just to the south and south-west of Nairobi in Kajiado and Narok Districts live the Maasai-speaking people. They overspill the Kenya-Tanzania border and a significant proportion lives in the United Republic of Tanzania. The Maasai are the most famous herders of East Africa and are linguistically grouped as Plains Nilotes. They are related to the Turkana, the Teso, the Karamojong, the Jie, the Kuman, the Dobo, the Kuku and the Kakwa. This chapter examines Maasai traditional medicine and, in particular, its role in the health care of the community. Initially the various specializations of Maasai traditional healers are outlined and then the concept of disease causation among the Maasai is probed. The final part of the chapter provides empirical data on Maasai traditional healers. These data were obtained from fieldwork in Narok District between 1989 and 1992.

Maasai Traditional Medicine

Traditional medicine is deeply rooted among the Maasai who have wide knowledge of herbal medicines which they use in treating humans and also for conditioning and treating livestock. In traditional Maasai society, herbal mixtures were used as digestives and/or excitants, especially by the *il murran* (warriors) preparing for raids (Table 8.1). For example, the herb *olkiloriti (Acacia nilotica)* was taken as a digestive, excitant and to prevent hunger and even thirst.

---

* Research for this chapter was supported by the International Development Research Centre (IDRC) Ottawa, Canada and the Rockefeller Foundation of New York. Some data in this chapter have already appeared in the authors's article in *Indigeous Knowledge and Developemnt Monitor* (Sindiga, 1994).

HolfordWalker recorded the following uses of the herb, *olkiloriti*:

> The Maasai state that neither fatigue nor fear, hunger nor thirst are felt after this drug is taken for sometime and that the *moran* always used to take it before going on raids (1951:1).

In short, herbal medicines pervaded many aspects of Maasai life in the past.

The Maasai refer to trees and shrubs collectively as *olcani* (pl. *ilkeek*) which also refers to woodfuel and medicine (Jacobs, 1963; Mol, 1978). The term *olcani* covers all medicine but it is specifically a reference to medicine extracted from plants.

Among the Maasai, trees and shrubs hold certain ritual significance in addition to providing shade for various social gatherings. Trees are so important that:

> only the wood, bark and leaves of trees may be used in certain purification ceremonies (*naipok*) to avert supernatural misfortune. Trees and shrubs are thus especially good, and their special ritual value . . . is closely associated with certain notions of Maasai cosmology (Jacobs, 1963:16).

Herbal medicines are used in a variety of circumstances. For this reason, nearly all the parts of a medicinal plant are used at one time or other.

> There are herbs, barks and roots which are boiled in soup and drunk to keep the stomach and the blood in good condition and there are those which are drunk when one is ill. There are also drugs derived from trees and shrubs for the cure of diseases such as gonorrhoea, stomach troubles, and infections connected with throat, pain in the sides (ribs), teeth, problems connected with pregnancy, eye infections, children's diseases, colds, swollen legs and painful joints, etc. (Sankan, 1971:60-61).

The Maasai procure treatment for numerous medical conditions in traditional medicine. It is the duty of every Maasai youth to learn the medicinal value of herbs as he or she grows up (Sankan, 1971). Traditionally, young boys are assigned the task of looking after small stock (goats and sheep) around the homesteads. In the process, they pick up knowledge on herbal medicines used in the home. Girls acquire their knowledge of herbal medicines from their mothers and grandmothers with whom they spend a lot of time (Sindiga, 1994). This explains partly why traditional medicine is entrenched in Maasai life. In brief, belief in the efficacy of traditional medicine, high levels of illiteracy in the society and the inaccessibility of health care all contribute to perpetuate Maasai beliefs in traditional medicine.

Table 8.1: Some herbal medicines and drugs used by the Maasai

Maasai name of herb	Botanical name	Part used	Condition it is used to treat	Mode of application
emokotan	*Albizzia anthelminthica*	branch wood; bark	medicinal (worms); (used by all Maasai) excitant	oral
enchaniangashe	—	roots	excitant; digestive	oral
endoroniki	—	roots	excitant; stimulant	not stated
engataru or *enongomani*	*Croton zambesieus*	branch wood; bark	excitant, digestive (used by morans)	Oral
engelinyei	*Rhoicissus eythrodes*	tuber root	excitant	oral
engelinyei	—	fibre liquid	medicinal (for wounds)	applied on wound
engoduai	—	berries; branch wood	excitant; medicinal; purgative	oral
olangungui	—	root tuber	excitant (morans only)	oral
oldimigomi	*Pappea cappensis*	wood; bark	digestive, stimulant (morans/elders use)	oral
olerai	*Acacia seyal*	bark; wood	stimulant; medicinal (fever, induce vomit) (morans only use)	oral
oljaninyuki	*Embella kilimandscharica*	bark	purgative; excitant; (morans only use)	oral
olkiloriti	*Acacia nilotica*	bark; roots	digestive; excitment; quench thrist; prevent hunger (wounded worriors)	oral
olkinyei	*Maba*	branch wood; bark	mild excitant; digestive; medicinal (for spleen)	oral
olkirenyi	—	bark; leaves	stimulant; mild excitant medicinal (colds, coughs,	oral

			medicinal (colds, coughs, fever) (elders/morans use it)	
olkitolosua	*Myrica kilimanshuarica*	root wood; root bark	stimulant; excitant (morans only use it)	oral
olkojyuk	—	roots	excitant	oral
olkonyeli	—	roots	stimulants, digestive; general tonic	not stated
olodua	*Maesa lanciolata*	roots	medicinal; excitant; stimulant; purgative	not stated
olokorododai	—	roots	digestive; flavour (mainly used by elders)	oral
osokonoi	.*Cassia*	bark; berries; root bark	excitant; medicinal; (malaria, coughs, colds)	oral
os sugurtuti or *ol dinai*	*Cissus* quadrangularis	branches	excitant	oral
Seketet (ngaita kik)	—	berries	purgative; excitant	oral

Maasai Traditional Healers

Although the basic knowledge of traditional medicine is almost universal among the Maasai, there are professional healers (*ilabaak;* sing. *olbaani*) in the society. Ordinarily, a sick person would be given treatment at home. When he failed to respond to the treatment the elders consult one another and take the patient to a professional healer. This means that a patient goes to a healer only after the illness has persisted for sometime. The healer would diagnose the problem through divination and other techniques and then provide the relevant medicine. This work is done by the *oloiboni* or *laibon* (pl. *oloibonok*), which concept is explained below.

---

* These data are from Holford-Walker (1951). The botanical names of some of the acacia species have been updated using Bogdan and Pratt (1974) and may not appear as in the original source.

Maasai traditional healers have several specializations (Table 8.2). However, as in other African communities, most healers combine two or more specializations. A Maasai medicineman (*oloiboni*) is a herbalist, diviner, spiritualist, fortune teller and ritual expert who provides supernatural guidance to the community (Mol, 1978; Fosbrooke, 1938). The term *iloibonok* tends to be an all-encompassing concept for Maasai medicinemen. Because of the significance of the *oloiboni* in Maasai ritual and healing life it is imperative to explain the concept in detail.

Table 8.2: Major categories of Maasai traditional healers (*Ilabaak*)

Category	Maasai name	Role
Diviner, spiritualist, fortune teller	*oloiboni* (pl. *iloibonok*)	divination, foretelling, ritual expert, medicineman
Herbalist	*enkaria*	various conditions
Traditional birth attendant (TBA)	*enkaitoyioni* (pl. *inkaitoyiok*)	antenatal, perinatal and postnatal care
Surgeon (female)	—	clitoridectomy
Surgeon (male)	*enkamuratani* or *olamuratani* *oltorobani*	circumcision
Bone-setter	*oloenani looloik*	fractures, wounds
Dentist	—	removes bad (malformed) teeth from infants and children

Following the work of Fosbrooke (1938) and my fieldwork in Narok, it would appear that there are three categories of Maasai *laibon* based on seniority and geographical coverage with regard to scale of operation (Figure 8.1). The first category comprises a traditional healer practising in his local community and consulting with individuals in the immediate vicinity of his home. He may be considered a private practitioner. His duties involve treating various diseases including infertility and securing infidelity in wives. Such a healer is paid fees by the individuals who consult him.

The second category emerges when, as the reputation of the private practitioner increases on account of the quality of his work, he takes on more functions. In addition to serving the the role of private practitioner, he is consulted by deputations representing a Maasai group which may be a clan, a section or any such group. The healer may then be regarded as a consultant and his duties expand to include providing charms to warriors for success in war, providing charms to confer immunity against disease, and even providing charms for sufficient rainfall (Fosbrooke, 1938). (Traditionally the *il murran* consulted a *laibon* on the advisability of a planned raid).

The third category of a Maasai *laibon* is what Fosbrooke (1938) calls a superintendent or chief medicineman (Figure 8.1). A superintendent combines the duties of a private practitioner and consultant and, in addition, conducts ceremonies such as circumcision and warrior promotion which affect the whole tribe. Conceptually, the three categories/stages in the developemnt of Maasai medicinemen may be seen along the same continuum. They reveal a nested hierarchy of development from a small time practitioner with limited functions and dealing with individuals in a localized area, to a renowned figure with diverse functions at a larger geographical scale at the level of the entire tribe (Figure 8.2).

Figure 8.1: Stages in the development of a Maasai medicineman

Private practitioner *Functions*	**Consultant** *Functions*	**Superintendent (chief medicineman)** *Functions*
• cures sickness • cures infertility • secures infidelity in wives • consulted only by individual patients at a fee	• functions identical to private practitioner • provides charms for success in war • sufficient rainfall, immunity against disease • consulted by a deput-ation of a Maasai group	• does the roles of practitioner and consultant • conducts ceremonies affecting whole tribe e.g. circumcision, warrior promotion. • Supernatural guidance.

SOURCE: Data from *A Sociological Survey of the Maasai of Tanganyika Territory* Compiled by H.A. Fosbrooke (1938).

The chief medicineman was traditionally the acknowledged *laibon* of the tribe or group of sections (Fosbrooke, 1938). In fact, it would appear that each Maasai section had its own *laibon* whose position was hereditary. However, distant relatives could work as private practitioners and consultants. Contrary to some colonial government accounts that a *laibon* was a paramount chief, the evidence suggests the contrary. A *laibon* was only chief priest considered to be the religious head of the Maasai (Storrs-Fox, 1930). In this role, the Maasai considered the *laibon*

> to be capable of controlling . . unseen forces; he is the intermediary between themselves and the supernatural. His blessing will assure prosperity, his charms and rituals can alleviate an existing calamity, and his power of foretelling the future enables steps to be taken to ward off an impeding catastrophe (Fosbrooke, 1938:26).

Iloibonok's power of divining, foretelling the future and cursing those breaching a taboo made the holder of the office very influential. According to some informants, *iloibonok* were respected and even adored. People took property to the *laibon* to make him strong. A *laibon*, in traditional Maasai society, is said to have been stronger and more influential than the chief of today. This is why the *iloibonok* were almost automatically regarded as leaders and assumed the roles.

The great influence the *iloibonok* held in the traditional Maasai society is not entirely surprising. In the south east Asian state of Bali, the power to communicate with the supernatural on behalf of the group propels an individual healer to higher socio-economic status and to a position of authority in society (McCauley, 1984:167-172). This would create a state of inequality in which the healers with such power become more prosperous than healers in other categories.

Fig. 8.2: Nested hierarchy of Maasai medicinemen

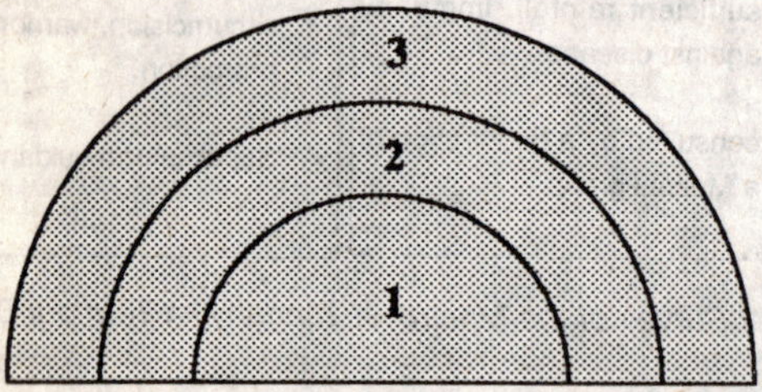

1. = Local medicineman consulted by individuals within the immediate community.

1,2 = Local medicineman with a reputation beyond the immediate community and geographical area: covers a wider group e.g. clan or sub-section. Consulted by local people and others from beyond.

1,2,3 = Chief medicineman shouldering functions of 1 and 2; in addition he oversees ceremonies and other duties for the section or whole tribe. In popular usage, the term laibon refers to the medicineman at this level. Only the laibon can offer supernatural guidance to the group.

Concept of Disease Causation Among the Maasai

Maasai beliefs on what causes disease are not well articulated (Olenja and Kratz, 1986:100). The following account is pieced together from data from field interviews and reference to documentary sources.

The Maasai hold disease aetiologies similar to those of the Luo (see Chapter 6). Disease/illness (*emueyian; pl. imueyiaritin*) is believed to emanate from the environment via food, water, hygiene, sex and weather changes. Informants cited examples such as eating a dead cow's meat whereby such meat may be contaminated with certain diseases, for example, anthrax (*entemelua*) and blackwater. Malaria (*oltikana*) usually follows the period of rainy weather and is believed to be caused naturalistically. Informants also cited sexually transmitted diseases as coming from male-female sexual contact. However, it could not be established whether this view was held in Maasai tradition or it had been acquired from modern health sources.

The Maasai also recognize the diseases spread by wildlife; for example, a calving wildebeeste leaves its foetal membranal substances on the grass which are contaminated with the virus which causes malignant catarrh fever (*engeea oinkat*). This disease is deadly to cattle.

Also, certain diseases may be caused by people through witchcraft or evil spirits from the living dead. This is taken to be the case when a couple loses children frequently through death. The same is true if livestock die frequently. Such conditions are attended to by the traditional healers.

Poisoning through herbs is quite common among the Maasai. The so-called black magic is seldom practised in the community; in fact, several informants insisted that the Maasai did not have witches and wizards who prawl or run at night. Whatever witchcraft the Maasai may have is claimed not to be indigenous to them (Storrs-Fox, 1930). (Storrs-Fox attributed the origins of Maasai witchcraft to the Kikuyu of Nyeri or the Meru. However, it has not been possible to verify these claims).

Certainly, evil eye (*mbusurek*) is quite prevalent among the Maasai. Sankan (1971;60) does not understand the scourge of evil eye and he believes that it is nothing more than conjouring tricks. He labels the healers who treat the condition as tricksters and appears to be unaware of evil mystical power so effectively described by Mbiti:

> There is mystical power which causes people to walk on fire, to lie on thorns or nails, to send curses or harm, including death from a distance, to change into animals (lycanthropy), to spit on snakes and cause them to split open and die; . . . power to make inanimate objects turn into biologically living creatures . . . (1969: 197-198).

Witches and sorcerers use power derived from evil spirits to cause illness. *Mbusurek* is a perfect example of the workings of evil power to cause constipation and ultimate death if not attended to quickly by the medicineman.

Other diseases may come about as a result of breaching taboo or from cursing by ancestors. However, these conditions can be handled by the traditional healers.

A Survey of Maasai Ethnomedical Practice

This section provides further data on Maasai traditional medical practice. The data were collected in three sub-locations occupied by the Maasai in Narok District, namely Naroosura, Olmesutie and Ololturot (Table 8.3). In all, field interviews were conducted with 90 traditional healers (Naroosura, 55; Olmesutie, 10; and Ololturot, 25) using a questionnaire.

The basic data on the numbers of healers and the population of the study sublocations are given on Table 8.3. The sub-locations represented here were fairly sparsely populated with densities ranging from seven to 10 persons per square kilometre in 1991. Table 8.3 shows that there are many traditional healers among the Maasai: The ratio of healers to the population was 1:40 for Olmesutie and 1:56 for Naroosura. This suggests greater availability of the healers to the populations that consume their services.

Profile of Maasai healers

On average, Maasai traditional healers appeared to be older people. Their mean age was 56 years with the median at 57 years (N= 89). Most Maasai healers (54%), were married with the rest (35% widowed). It is significant that single people, who, in this case are the "never-maaried", were not represented in Maasai traditional medicine.

On average, Maasai healers had stayed in practice for 22 years with a median of 23 years; this figure was 20 years for Ololturot, and Naroosura Sub-locations and 30 years in Olmesutie.

All the healers were asked to state their formal education background. Virtually all the Maasai healers were illiterate. Of the 80 healers who answered the question on education, only one person said he had atttended primary school.

In terms of religious affiliation, most (94%) of the healers (N=84) adhered to their own traditional religion. Only four per cent of the healers professed to be Christians. The issue of religion is related to education. In most parts of Kenya, the expansion of education went hand in hand with Christianity. It would appear that areas with few education opportunities also have little foreign religious influence. The Maasai nomadic lifestyle partly explains this phenomenon. During the long dry season, the Maasai have traditionally moved to places where they could obtain fodder and water for their livestock -school children must abandon their education to move with the livestock. Also, traditionally, Maasai men spent long periods in residence undergoing the rites of initiation, circumcision, warriorhood and finally marriage. At present most Maasai girls do not go to school, even those who do, abandon it soon afterwards to get married. It is common to find Maasai girls marrying in their middle teenage years before they are 20 years old.

Table 8.3: Aggregate numbers of traditional healers in Narok (1991)

Sublocation	Land area (km^2)	Estimated population, 1991**	Healers*	TBAs	All healers	Healer to population
Olmesutie	352	3,621	57	33	90	1:40
Naroosura	1,111	7,906	73	68	141	1:56
Ololturot	N/A	N/A	35	13	48	—

Notes: N/A - Not available. Ololturot is in Mosiro Location and the latter was subdivided after 1979.

* The figures include TBAs who also practised as herbalists

** The 1991 population was estimated on the base of the 1979 population assuming the national annual growth rate of 3.34% (Kenya, 1991).

Becoming a Maasai traditional healer

Maasai healers do not get formal training for their vocation. Instead, the healing skill is gained through informal training or is inherited from family members. A notable proportion of the sample comprising 40 per cent of the healers (N = 87) served for periods as either apprentices or learner-observers with practising healers. Only a very small percentage (3%) claimed that their practice was God-given. Presumably, such people were required by their ancestral spirits to practise traditional medicine. This is usually done through dreams, revelations or sickness.

Patient caseload

The healers were asked to state the number of clients they had seen over the week prior to the interview. The mean as well as median number of patients was two. Perhaps the reason for this relatively low percentage owes to the fact that the Maasai people know a wide range of traditional herbs which they utilize and therefore see a specialist only when they fail to obtain a cure at home. Also, certain diseases increase or diminish in prevalence according to season - usually increasing in the rainy periods. Other tasks such as circumcision take place only at certain times of the year, that is August and December.

In terms of time sharing between traditional medicine and other activities, 45 per cent of the traditional healers acknowledged traditional medicine as a full time vocation (N = 88). For the majority, representing 55 per cent, traditional medical practice was a part-time activity. However, even those who claimed to be full-time healers also kept large numbers of livestock which were tended by their family members. Thus, in reality, there were very few full-time healers who would be said to derive their entire livelihood from traditional medicine.

Maasai traditional healers treat many conditions ranging from the whole gamut of medical and social conditions including bad dreams, "dream" walking, evil spirits, diarrhoea, infertility and general body weakness, to fortune telling.

In terms of medicines, Maasai healers use a large variety of herbs which are present in their surrounding. They also utilize honey and animal fat in the treatment process.

Majority of the healers (94%) collected and prepared the herbs themselves; they collected the herbs from the bush both within their environment and from distant places. They do not plant any herbs, but rely heavily on the rich floral landscape which they occupy.

Fees payment

Maasai healers are paid fees; only a negligible proportion of the healers claimed it does not receive any fees. The fees is now increasingly paid in cash or both in cash and materials and only eight per cent of the healers interviewed received fees only in kind (N=84). This trend reflects the extent of the monetarization of the Maasai economy and the increasing significance of cash even among the pastoral peoples.

When asked about the time when fees payment was demanded in relation to the course of therapy, the majority of healers (65%) said they were paid "after treatment". No healer charged fees before treatment and a small proportion (8%) received it on the commencement of treatment (N = 88). It is to be noted that a significant proportion of the healers (20%) received payment after their clients had obtained cure.

When the healers were asked about the basis of the level of fees they demanded, the responses were mixed. Some 31 per cent said that the level of fees depended on the ability of the client to pay, 35 per cent based it on the nature and complexity of the illness, and 33 per cent asked a constant fee for all conditions

(N = 81).

Data on fees charged for a number of diseases were quite variable. The acutal amounts paid really depended on the individual healer and the client. The clients who paid in kind usually gave livestock; however, the healers accepted pieces of meat or even beer in lieu of a live animal. Such charges were difficult to quantify or compare with another location.

Consultation venue

Maasai healers do not have clinics. Their clients go to see them at home. However, the majority of the healers (72%) did not provide special overnight accommodation for their clients (N = 85). This was probably because most of the clients came from within the healers' own sub-locations. Only 9 per cent of the healers (N = 90) said that they attended to clients who came from outside Narok District.

Record keeping and patient referrals

Nearly all the Maasai healers interviewed were illiterate. It is perhaps not surprising that none of them kept a record on the clients (N = 87).

The healers were also asked to provide data on patient referrals. The issue here is whether the healers made patient referrals to fellow healers and to biomedical facilities and personnel. Referrals to other traditional healers were frequent representing 44 per cent of the interviewees (N = 88). The majority of the healers (56%) did not make any such referrals. However, the healers sent their patients to the modern medicinemen. The majority (55%) said that they did so.

However, biomedical practitioners did not refer their patients to traditional healers. It is the patients themselves who made the decision to see traditional healers after visiting the facility. Maasai healers believe that certain diseases can best be handled in the hospital — complicated fractures, venereal disease, measles, poliomyelitis, tuberculosis, brucellosis, pneumonia and meningitis. At the same time the healers noted that certain diseases can only be cured in traditional medicine; infertility, mental disorders, genital worms, misfortunes and evil spirits.

Cooperation between traditional healers and biomedical personnel

One of the objectives of the study was to establish the possibilities of involving traditonal healers in cooperative relationships with health personnel in primary health care. When asked on whether they thought that there should be such relationships, the majority of the healers (84%) answered in the negative (N= 84). Only a small minority representing 16 per cent of the healers thought such cooperation as necessary.

The Maasai healers were not willing to get training in any aspect of modern medicine either. Out of a total of 85 healers who answered the question, a resounding 98 per cent (the majority) dismissed training in modern health care (N = 85).

Conclusion

This chapter has shown the importance of traditional medicine in the life of the Maasai. Also, it has formulated a conceptual framework of analyzing Maasai traditional healers. This framework provides for a nested hierarchy of development of the healer from a small-time practitioner with limited functions in a geographically restricted area, to a renowned figure operating both socially and areally in wider space.

Through the use of empirical data collected in Narok District, the chapter provides detailed information on Maasai traditional medical practitioners including their training and specializations. It is clear that training for certain areas of traditional medicine is difficult owing to the mystery that shrouds the acquisition of such skills. Perhaps this is why family inheritance of the practice is prevalent in many communities. In the Maasai case, families of the *iloibonok* tend to be well known.

This chapter has also revealed that traditonal healers make cross-referrals to biomedical people, but the reverse is not so. This may be an impediment to utilizing the potential manpower in traditional medicine in respect of primary health care (see chapter 1). Successful cooperative relationships should stem from an appreciation of the strengths and weaknesses of any system of medicine and its mutual respect which could create an environment of cooperation. It should also be noted that Maasai healers were not enthusiastic about working together with official health care providers. This is partly because the Maasai pastoral culture, especially in the drier part of Narok, remains more or less intact. Nevertheless, the incipient changes taking place are likely to affect Maasai traditional medicine, gradually.

REFERENCES

Bogdan, A.V. and D.J. Pratt. 1974. *Common Acacias of Kenya*. Nairobi: Government Printer.

Fosbrooke, H.A. 1938. "A Sociological Survey of the Maasai of Tanganyika Territory." File No. DC/NRK/6/1/1. Kenya National Archives.

Holford-Walker, A. F. 1951. "Herbal Medicines and Drugs Used by the Maasai." Political Records – Miscellaneous — Narok District. File No. DC/NRK/3/1. Kenya National Archives.

Jacobs, A. H. 1963. "*The Pastoral Maasai of Kenya: Report of Anthropological Field Research*. London: Ministry of Overseas Development.

Kenya, Government of 1991. *Economic Survey 1991*. Nairobi: Central Bureau of Statistics.

Mbiti, J. S. 1969. *African Religions and Philosophy*. London: Heinemann.

McCauley, A. P. 1984. "Healing as a Sign of Power and Status in Bali." *Social Science and Medicine* 18 No. 2: 167-172.

Mol, F. 1978. *Maa: A Dictionary of the Maasai Language and Folklore — English-Maasai*. Nairobi: Marketing and Publishing.

Olenja, J. M. and C. Kratz. 1968. "*Medicine and Health. Narok District Socio-Cultural Profile Draft Report*. Nairobi: Ministry of Planning and National Development and University of Nairobi. pp. 95-104.

Sankan, S.S. 1971. *The Maasai*. Nairobi: East African Literature Bureau.

Sindiga, I. 1994. "Indigenous (medical) Knowledge of the Maasai." *Indigenous Knowledge and Development Monitor* 2 No. 1: 16-18.

Storrs-Fox, D. 1930 "Further Notes on the Maasai of Kenya Colony." *Journal of Royal Anthropological Institute* 60: 447-465.

Chapter 9

GUSII TRADITIONAL MEDICINE*

Isaac Sindiga

This chapter outlines Gusii traditional medicine and highlights the community's concept of disease causation and the practitioners in this medical system. It aims to show that the gap between the accessibility and availability of modern health services and the demand for these services is filled by traditional medicine.

Background

The Gusii-speaking people are part of the Bantu group in western Kenya and are related to the Luyia, Suba and the Kuria. The Gusii-speakers are called Abagusii, (sing. Omogusii) and their country, which comprises Nyamira and Kisii districts (area, 2,196 Km[1]) is known as Gusii. Their language is Ekegusii. Living at the south-western end of the Kenya highlands, the Abagusii were projected to number some 1,559,000 people in 1993 (Kenya, 1989: 13). The history of their settlement in Gusii has been done elsewhere (Ochieng', 1974; Bogonko, 1977).

The Abagusii are a culturally homogeneous group whose population appears to have grown rapidly from 225,000 people in 1948 to 519,000 in 1962 and 675,000 in 1969 to 971,000 in 1979 and 1,146,000 in 1989 (Uchendu and Anthony, 1975: 14-15; Kenya, 1991:32). This population explosion, resulting from natural increase, gives Gusii the distinction of being one of the most densely populated rural areas by world standards. The average crude density is about 700 persons per square kilometre with some areas exceeding 900 persons.

The Gusii Medical System

The Abagusii have an elaborate traditional medical system with a variety of practitioners, specializations, pharmacopoeia and medical paraphernalia. This

* Data used in this chapter were collected with financial support from the Rockefeller Foundation of New York for the period 1989-1993.

system exists side by side with modern medicine. It is used almost exclusively when measles (*omokururo* or *ekanyamoguku*) appears in children. In fact, the Abagusii do not take measles victims to the hospital before the rash appears. Other conditions for which the Abagusii do not seek modern medicine are evil eye (ebibiriria); and *orosao rwa abana* (infantile diarrhoea) (Nyamwaya, 1986) which they believe is caused by abnormal development of milk teeth (*ebisara*).

The foregoing indicates that the Abagusii make a distinction between diseases or conditions which have to be drawn to biomedicinal attention and those that are preserved for traditional medicine. How is the distinction made? Who makes the distinction? Why is the distinction made? Does therapy-selection follow the distinction? To understand this phenomenon, one must delve into the disease aetiologies of the culture concerned.

Disease Causation and Therapy Choice*

The Abagusii do not distinguish between disease, illness or misfortune. Although diseases (*amarwaire*; sing. *oborwaire*) are believed to be caused in a number of ways; when a person falls sick or even dies, the Abagusii tend to tag a human-induced cause, especially witchcraft, to the case. Equally important are the supernatural causes of disease.

In the realm of the supernatural, diseases may be caused by ancestral spirits (*chisokoro*; sing. *esokoro*). It is the duty of the living *omogusii* to lubricate relationships between them and the departed ancestors. This takes the form of livestock sacrifices, usually cattle, sheep, goats and chicken. In normal circumstances, once a father has offered sacrifice to the *chisokoro*, the son or sons need not do it. But the grandsons are obliged to do so. Failure to remember the ancestors may lead to the punishment of family members. They may remain poor or they could be afflicted with ill health and sometimes death.

The anger of *chisokoro* may be expressed through evil spirits (*ebirecha*; sing. *ekerecha*). If, for example, a father is not buried properly on his death, his spirits could become angry and affect a family member. Such would show themselves in madness (*ebarimo*) or make a woman barren/infertile (*omogomba*; pl. *abagomba*) or make a child to contract epilepsy (*endurume*). A father's proper burial consists of first slaughtering a cockerel (*etwoni*), followed by a he-goat (*egoree*) after three days. After two to three months another *egoree* or *emingichi* (ram) is slaughtered to cleanse the home. At this stage, a surviving fertile widow may be

* My understanding of the concept of disease and illness among the Abagusii was illuminated and clarified by discussions with Omogaka Clement Nyandara and Mr. Wilfred Nyangesi both of Bonchari and retired church leader Abel Nyakundi Onchoke of Kiogoro, Nyaribari Chache.

inherited by another man for the purpose of continuing procreation in the dead man's name.

There are a number of other causes of *ebirecha*. These include spotting a python, killing a person, or killing *omogere* (a *Jaluo*). The affected family is expected to go to a diviner (*omoragori*) to find out the underlying cause and then take required action, usually taking herbal medicine and sacrifice. In the case of killing a person, a black sheep is usually slaughtered. This is believed to chase away the evil spirits.

The Abagusii also believe that witchcraft is responsible for certain medico-social problems. These include mental disturbance (*ebarimo*), infertility (*obogomba*), and developing a chronic wound *(rikwege*; pl. *amakwege*). Another problem resulting from bewitching (*ogokonwa*) is epilepsy (*endurume*) and evil eye (*ebibiriria*).

Both witches (*abarogi;* sing. *omorogi*) and sorcerers (*abanyamosira*) are well known within Gusii society. Witches are particularly feared among the Abagusii and their actions appear to be motivated by jealousy (Le Vine and Le Vine, 1966:95-97). Sometimes *abanyamosira* also act as healers to deal with the effects of witchcraft in society.

Certain diseases are believed to be inherited (*ororeria*). Such diseases may be passed along the lineage line to the offspring. A good example is *enyaini* or *endonge* (liver cirrhosis). The liver enlarges and hardens ultimately developing a wound. Chronic *enyani* causes oedema of the feet. At this stage, a person will die. *Enyaini* is treated by Gusii traditional medicine.

Another condition which is believed to be inherited is *ebarimo* (mental disturbance). However, passing diseases along the lineage line need not be direct. (i.e. parent to offspring). The problem could have existed among the living-dead members of the family especially grandparents.

Another cause of disease and ill health among the Abagusii is breaching taboos, taking perjured oaths, and sexual offences, especially adultery. These sets of offences draw the anger of ancestral spirits which administer punishment. Adultery is punished by *amasangia*. The latter is the supernatural punishment against the infidelity of a wife. The actions of an adulterous woman affect her husband and children and may cause death. Men's extramarital relations with married women is also held in check by *amasangia* (Le Vine and Le Vine, 1966).

Finally, the Abagusii believe that disease may be caused in a naturalistic way. *Enyamo* or *omwaga* is a problem of bad air which attacks children and adults. The primary symptom is an allergy demonstrated by swelling all over the body. It is believed that changes in seasons may bring bad air from distant lands. The Luo have a similar condition called *yamo* (See Chapter 6 and 7).

In general, naturalistic diseases are picked in the environment. They are amenable to herbal remedies. Such include asthma *(ekeera or egekuba egeku*), splenomegally (*endwari ya inda*), malaria (*esosera*) and diarrhoea (*orosao*).

Although this is an attempt to delineate clear disease aetiologies held by the Abagusii, such classification is only useful for analysis and greater comprehension of the culture's conception of disease and illness. In reality, the Abagusii:

> maintain contradictory explanations of disease, one of which views disease as punishment for sexual, aggressive, property and ritual offences, while the other more frequently used, blames it on the unwarranted malevolence of others (Le Vine and Le Vine, 1966:104).

This is what makes the Abagusii

> pragmatic about treatment and will try anything that promises help and that has the faith of someone they respect. When one remedy fails, they try another, running through injections,... tablets, sacrifice and sorcery with no feeling of inconsistency (Le Vine and Le Vine, 1966:93).

Nyamwaya (1986:102-103) notes that the Abagusii first seek meaning in the physical causation or what he calls the "how" explanation of illness. Only in cases of mental ailments or chronic disease is a "why" explanation sought. According to him, there are two categories of causes which are attributed to the "why" explanation, namely interpersonal (witchcraft, curse or breaching of a taboo or custom) and spiritual (ancestors). The interpersonal factors are "the stresses, guilt and emotional disturbances which are the consequences of sins or crimes committed by the patient or his fellow men". (p. 102). He concludes that

> the "why" type of causation deals with social responsibility for an illness. An individual who deviates from the social norms cherished by the community will bring punishment on himself or his family (pp. 102-103).

Thus, the Abagusii look to the various possibilities of causes when an illness strikes. They may utilize modern medicine together with herbal remedies. The latter are to protect them against evil people. Simultaneously, they may sacrifice an animal just in case the problem comes from the supernatural. In other words, the Abagusii make an open-ended search for treatment within the medical systems which are accessible and available until the disease/illness is cured. Rather than providing a key to simple and swift selection of a medical system, the diverse disease aetiologies tend to provide the basis for the uncertainty as to the actual cause of a given illness. The result is a rather diffuse pattern of therapy- seeking behaviour.

Practitioners of Gusii Traditional Medicine

The Gusii traditional medical system comprises several specialists. These are listed in Table 9.1. The basic traditional healer is *omonyamete*, literally herbal dispenser. He or she is found everywhere and usually dispenses herbal remedies for conditions that are believed to be natural. The healer who deals in love charms is called *omoebia*.

Another category of healers is the diviner (*omoragori*). *Abaragori* usually unravel the cause of a given condition, especially one emanating from either supernatural or human-induced causes. After diagnosing the cause, *omoragori* also advises on a course of action to avert the problem. There is also a category of people who foretell the future through prophecy called *ababani*, who are rather like fortune-tellers. There is also another category of healers comprising traditional birth attendants (*abarabi*). These provide a variety of services including antenatal, prenatal and postnatal care and counsel expectant mothers on the appropriate foods to eat (Omburo, 1988:47). *Abarabi* are significant in the Gusii society because of the high demand for children. Gusii men and women share a "strong desire for offspring" (Le Vine and Le Vine, 1966:111). Among the Abagusii, childlessness is believed to be a sin-consequence for perjured oaths, punishment for breaching a taboo or custom; and displeasure of the ancestors for failing to appease them.

Table 9.1: Major categories of Gusii traditional healers

Category		Function
Singular	**Plural**	
omonyamete	*abanyamete*	herbalist
omoragori	*abaragori*	diviner
omoriori	*abarioti*	one who unearths magic/ witchcraft materials and medicine. "Witch smeller" (Le Vine and Le Vine, 1966:84).
omorabi	*abarabi*	traditional birth attendant
omobari	*ababari*	surgeon
omosari	*abasari*	circumcisor
omoromeki	*abaromeki*	one who performs localized blood letting to relieve pain.
omoebia	*abaebia*	dealer in love medicines;
omwati	*abati*	undertakes autopsies
omonyibi embura	*abanyibi embura*	rain maker
omokireki	*abakireki*	one who uses medicines to prevent disease and misfortune.
omobani	*ababani*	one who foretells the future.
omonyamosira	*abanyamosira*	sorcerer.

Sources: Nyamwaya, 1986: 107-109; 1992:8

Perhaps the most remarkable feature of Gusii traditional medicine is surgery.

The surgeons (*ababari*) are particularly known for the surgical procedure called craniotomy or head trephining which really is the opening of the brain case to relieve pressure which causes headaches in brain tumours (Thairu, 1975:87). The *omobari* has deep knowledge of the human body, suturing and antisepsis, essential for his surgical work. Such specialization is also well known among the Meru, Kuria and Marakwet (Nyamwaya, 1992:12).

Other specialists in related areas are *abasari* (circumcisors), *abati* who drain abscesses and undertake autopsies and *abaromeki* who puncture a part of the body to release pressure thereby relieving pain. Male circumcisors operate on boys whereas the women conduct clitoridectomy. Female circumcision is still very much a revered tradition among the Abagusii.

As explained above, witchcraft is quite feared among the Abagusii. Witches use certain magical materials to inflict suffering on their targets. However, such harm can be done by *abanyamosira* or *abanyanabi* (sorcerers). Sometimes the sorcerers can be used as healers. In this capacity, they utilize their medicines to retaliate against witchcraft or to protect a family from it by performing a protective ritual called *okoosia* (Le Vine and Le Vine, 1966:98). Also, witches usually consult *abanyamosira* to obtain protective medicine to counter the effort.

Also, a special healer called *omoriori* uses medicine to sniff out and unearth the magic or witchcraft materials and medicines causing illness. Medicines neutralize their potency and render them useless. *Omoriori* is sometimes dubbed a "witch-smeller" (Le Vine and Le Vine, 1966:84), although he works only to remove the paraphernalia of witchcraft rather than smelling the witches themselves.

Profile of a Gusii traditional healer

Some 10 kilometers to the south-west of Kisii town along the Kisii-Kilgoris road at Boburia village, Boronyi Sub-location, Nyaribari Chache, lives Pastor (retired) Abel Nyakundi Onchoke. Born in 1901, Nyakundi earned a diploma in evangelism at the Seventh Day Adventist Training School, Kamagambo, in 1942 after two years' study. He was made a pastor in 1948 and retired in 1975 after working for 27 years. I interviewed Nyakundi during September 1989 at his home.

Nyakundi is a herbalist but he mixes this with Christian prayer. His father was a traditional healer working as *omoriori* and the mother was a diviner. This background enabled Nyakundi to work as an apprentice to his parents as he grew up. He said that he inherited the knowledge of the treatment of various medical conditions from his mother. He intimated, however, that the knowledge of certain herbal medicines is revealed to him by God. Nyakundi believes that faith and herbal remedies work together to control a disease or illness.

After retiring from his religious duties, Nyakundi took to full-time work as a herbalist. He had practised as a traditional healer for 20 years suggesting that he combined his pastoral work with herbal treatment for some time. When I interviewed him in 1989, he had four assistants – his wife, son and two grandsons. The assistants were on a training programme and had mastered various herbs used in treating different conditions.

Nyakundi listed about 40 diseases that he was able to treat among them women infertility (*abakungu bateneine*) and also said that he could provide medicine to women who gave birth to female children consecutively to get a male child and vice versa. Other diseases he handles are diabetes, hypertension, nose bleeding, chronic headache, asthma (*egekuba egeku or ekeera*) gonorrhoea (*enyamosono* or *enyamorero*), boils (*esamusamu*), abortion and premature births, poisoning (*esumu*), abdominal pains in women during or after the menses (*chinkegeto chia omoiseke)*, chronic wound (*rikwege* or *esiri*). In addition he provides herbal remedies to women who miss their menses.

Nyakundi kept a strict record of his patients. On average, he made consultations with 10 patients every week. His patient record showed the name of the client, place of origin, diagnosis, treatment/herbs administered or provided, the amount of fees paid and the balance to be paid in future. On consultation fees, Nyakundi said he charged inexpensively because of his belief that his knowledge of herbal medicines was a gift from God. He could not exploit it for profit.

The healer noted that many of his patients came to him after seeking treatment in modern facilities. This suggests that either the problem could not be handled successfully in biomedicine or the patients did not wait through the course of initial therapy before looking for an alternative (see Chapter 6).

During the week preceding our interview, Nyakundi had been consulted by patients suffering from infertility (women), asthma, malaria and amoeba. He treated women infertility with the roots of*moteoitimo* herbs, asthma with the leaves of *moteokebaki*, and amoeba with the leaves of *omonyantira* or *ekemwa*; however, malaria was treated with 22 different herbs.

Nyakundi collected herbal medications from the bush himself. Nevertheless, owing to his advancing age, his assistants had increasingly taken over the chore. Also, he noted that bushland was receding forcing him to walk long distances in search of the herbs. He had planted a few herbs which were very difficult to obtain.

*Discussion**

Pastor Nyakundi represents the contemporary workers in Gusii traditional medicine. Most of them are herbalists, other cadres are scattered widely apart. Both men and women practise Gusii medicine many of whom are older people, usually over 50 years of age. Gusii healers are experienced and each has practised for a median of 20 years. Again, most practitioners inherit the vocation from their family members and/or work as apprentices to practising healers. Unlike Nyakundi, most of the Gusii traditional healers practise medicine as a part-time activity cultivating their land holdings for food and/or cash crops.

A survey of traditional healers in Bonchari in 1993 showed that they attended to a median of four patients per week (c.f 10 for Nyakundi). They treated a large range of medical conditions with herbal remedies collected by the healers themselves. Most of the herbs were collected from the bush although many healers also planted some herbs.

Conclusion

This chapter has outlined the Abagusii concept of what causes disease, illness and misfortune. Although distinctive disease aetiologies are articulated, therapy-seeking behaviour tends to be pragmatic. The Abagusii move from one medical system to another without a sense of contradiction (c.f. Chapter 6).

Gusii traditional healers have many specializations; however, herbalists form the dominant group. The chapter has concluded with a profile of a Gusii traditional healer to add breadth to the discussion.

REFERENCES

Bogonko, S.N. 1977. *Christian Missionary Education and Its Impact on the Abagusii of Western Kenya 1909 to 1963*. Ph.D. Thesis, University of Nairobi.

Kenya, Government of. 1989. *Kisii District Development Plan 1989-1993*. Nairobi: Ministry of Planning.

__________. 1991. *Economic Survey 1991*. Nairobi: Central Bureau of Statistics.

Le Vine, R.A. and 1966. *Nyansongo: A Gusii Community in Kenya*. New York: John Wiley.

---

* Some of the data included in this section are based on interviews with 46 traditional healers in Suneka Division, Bonchari, Kisii District, during 1989.

Nyamwaya, D. 1986. "Health and Medicine" In *Kisii District Socio-Cultural Profile* edited by D. Nyamwaya. Nairobi: Ministry of Planning and National Development and University of Nairobi. pp. 100-111.

_______________. 1992. *African Indigenous Medicine: An Anthropological Perspective for Policy Makers and Primary Health Care Managers*. Nairobi: AMREF.

Ochieng', W. R. 1974. *A Precolonial History of the Gusii of Western Kenya A.D. 1500-1914*. Nairobi: East African Literature Bureau.

Thairu, K. 1975. *The African Civilization*. Nairobi: East African Literature Bureau.

Uchendu, V. C. and K. R. M. Anthony. 1975. *Agricultural Change in Kisii District, Kenya*. Nairobi: East African Literature Bureau.

Chapter 10

TRADITIONAL MEDICINE AMONG THE ABALUYIA

Simiyu Wandibba

This chapter discusses the traditional medical practices of the Abaluyia, a Bantu-speaking people, the majority of whom live in the Western Province of Kenya comprising Bungoma, Busia, Kakamega and Vihiga Districts. They overspill into the neighbouring Trans Nzoia District where they form a significant proportion of the population. Like other Kenyan communities, the Abaluyia are also to be found in all the major urban areas in the country. However, this chapter is concerned with the Abaluyia who live in Western Province.

The chapter starts by examining Luyia disease aetiologies which is the basis for discussing the Luyia therapeutic practices. Finally, the current state of traditional medicine among the Abaluyia is discussed.

Luyia Disease Aetiologies

Traditionally, the Abaluyia attributed disease and illness to multiple causes. They believed that illness may be caused by one of the following factors; the human factor, transgression against taboos, the spiritual factor, and environmental pollution. Let us look at each of these factors in turn, starting with the human factor.

Human factor

In traditional Luyia communities, there was widespread belief in the ability of some people to cause harm to others through evil designs. Such evil people employed either witchcraft (*bulosi* in Lubukusu or *ovulogi* in Olulogoli) to bring upon illness and other misfortunes on their perceived enemies. Witchcraft involved the use of special herbs and other medicines by *omulosi* (p. *balosi*) or *omulogi* (pl. *avalogi*) to cause illness. The witches (*balosi* or *avalogi*) employed different techniques to harm their intended victims, some of which were gender-specific. Witches used such methods as dancing naked in the homestead of the victim, collecting materials associated with the victims (personal effects such as clothing, hair, nails, excreta or soil taken from their footprints), hiding deadly medicine across the path of the victim or in his homestead, and causing the victim to run into danger. The naked dancers were both men and women. They performed their dances in the courtyard whilst singing in low tones. The dance consisted of jumping up and down, pointing the bare buttocks at the door of the victim or banging against it before suddenly dashing off. To achieve the desired effect, the dancer had to combine the dance and a spell cast on *kamaloko* (in Lubukusu). *Kamaloko* (sing. *liloko*) were roots or small pieces of bark over which a spell was uttered as they were being ritually tied). This kind of witchcraft caused the victim to suffer from headache and pain in the muscles.

The collection of objects from victims was done by both men and women; this was, of course, done secretly. To achieve the evil purpose, the witch had to tie them with certain poisonous or magically destructive roots (Wagner, 1970) known, among the Babukusu, as *kamalesi*, which is also the generic name for modern medicines. Once the collected materials and the poisonous roots had been tied in a small bundle (*liloko*), they were placed in some appropriate receptacle for protection as a spell was recited. The receptacle was then hidden in some damp soil near a river, stream or spring. This kind of witchcraft led to a slow wasting away of the victim's health (Wagner, 1970).

The act of causing harm on a person by hiding deadly medicines as well as causing the victims to run into danger, were only practised by male witches. In the latter method, people were made to fall victim of sudden accidents or mishaps such as snake-bites, attacks from wild animals, suicides, drowning, or falling from a tree and breaking one's limbs. Writing about this particular method of witchcraft, Wagner (1970) states that this technique involved killing a special kind of lizard or procuring an egg from the victim's homestead. These objects were then cut open and some *kamalesi* put inside.

> Then, without tying it, he hides the object at a place near which the intended victim will pass or over which he will step. While burying it there, he mutters a spell, specifying the kind of accident or death which he desires the victim to meet with . . . (Wagner, 1970;115).

The hiding of deadly medicines is done either in the homestead of the victim or at a spot over which the victim will pass. The medicines so buried emit their poison through the air to the victim. Because of their potency, these medicines cause instant death on their victims.

Those witchcraft techniques restricted to women included the throwing of *bilasila* (Lubukusu) and infecting the food of others. *Bilasila* comprised tiny objects such as hairs, bits of grass, beans, splinters of bones and so on (Wagner 1970), objects which were mysteriously transmitted from the witch into the body of her victim. Wagner (1970:116) states that,

> when these objects have entered the victim's body, they cause acute sickness, a swollen stomach and cramps accompanied by vomiting, an intense headache, hot temples and a generally feverish condition.

This kind of witchcraft was especially directed against children and involved putting certain particles, such as the hair of a dead fox or excreta of a hyena, secretly into the food of the victim. Some of these particles could cause immediate death while others simply brought about stomachache and vomiting.

Sorcery (*ovuvila*) was traditionally found only in Kakamega and Vihiga Districts. Sorcerers, *avavila* or *avafila* (sing. *ombila* or *omufila*), were believed to possess both destructive as well as protective magic. However, of concern in this section is the destructive magic. The *ombila's* lethal medicines consisted exclusively of herbs or roots which were either ground, dried, mixed, burnt or cooked. Among the Avalogoli, once the medicines had been prepared, they were put in a round, hair-shelled fruit locally known as *liveye* (pl. *amaveye*). According to Wagner:

> The most common technique employed by the *ambila* is to point a *liveye* filled with *ovuvila* at his intended victim, so that the opening of the *liveye* is directed towards him; at the same time he casts a bad look (*lihenza livi*) at him. The person at whom he had pointed the evil medicine . . . never sees the *liveye* itself, as the *ombila* always hides it in his fist (Wagner, 1970:134).

Because of their great potency, the *ombila's* medicines acted very fast on the victim; he became seriously ill within a few hours. He felt severe pain in the hand and limbs as well as aching in that side of the body on which the *ombila* passed.

Transgression against taboos

The second cause of disease in the traditional beliefs among the Abaluyia consisted of transgressions against taboos and ritual prohibitions. For instance, the Abaluyia observed a number of food taboos. People were prohibited from eating certain animals, both domestic and wild, as well as other food-stuffs. Whereas some of the food avoidances were based on clans others were observed on gender lines. Among the Bukusu, for example, each clan had at least one food taboo. However, many clans avoided eating the meat of the reed-buck (*esunu*) and that from *akhafu eng'enda* (a cow with a chequered design of brown and yellow colour). It was believed that if that kind of meat was eaten people would vomit and then become seriously ill.

Transgression against a food taboo inevitably made the victim suffer from some form of skin disease.

People who were in a state of ritual impurity were also believed to bring about illness and so had to be avoided until the performance of a lustration rite. In this category of people were widows, warriors who had killed their first enemy in battle, and women who had just given birth, especially to twins. It was believed that encounter with these people or sharing a meal with them before a purification rite had been performed for them would make the victim's skin yellow.

The spiritual factor

Another factor that could bring about illness and misfortune was displeasure from the ancestral spirits. The Abaluyia distinguished two types of ancestral spirits; the malevolent and benevolent. Among the Babukusu, the malevolent spirits were known as *bisieno* (sing. *sisieno*), while the benevolent ones were referred to as *bakuka* (sing. *omukuka*). The *bisieno* were believed to be the spirits of those people who, when alive, were witches or sorcerers. These spirits had one exclusive aim — to send misfortunes, sickness and death to their living relatives. They were responsible for such misfortunes as impotency, miscarriage and infertility in women. Illness such as epilepsy and madess were also ascribed to the work of *bisieno*.

On the other hand, the benevolent spirits acted as intercessors between the living and the supernatural power. Because of this belief, the living had to maintain a vertical relationship with their living dead. This they did through periodic sacrifices of livestock or poultry to the living dead. If the living ignored to maintain this relationship for one reason or another, the living dead could show their displeasure by causing disease, illness and misfortune. Sometimes, the *basambwa* also made certain demands on their living relatives through dreams and/or illness; for example, *omusambwa* who used to be a traditional healer or circumcisor might want one of the living relatives to inherit his art. If this revelation was ignored or remained undiagnosed, the dead person would enforce the message through inducement of illness. In fact, most instances of mental illness among the Abaluyia were believed to result from this phenomenon. However, illness induced in this way did not lead to death. Finally, *bakuka* could also induce illness if none of their living relatives was named after them. In this case, they showed their displeasure by causing discomfort to new-born babies or making such babies have diarrhoea. Again, such discomfort or illness did not lead to death.

The Abaluyia also believed that some illnesses such as epilepsy and some forms of madness were due to 'inheritance.' It was believed that such illnesses resulted from some curse and were passed on in families and clans.

Environmental pollution

The Abaluyia also ascribed some illnesses to environmental pollution; for example, Babukusu and Abatachoni believed that there were times when the air was contaminated and if such air was inhaled, the victim became ill. Air pollution occurred at the time of the first rains or when there was bloodshed. So, children were warned not to allow themselves to be made wet by the first rains as this would bring them down with influenza and common cold. On the other hand, when air had been contaminated by bloodshed, it was rendered harmless through sacrifice.

Finally, these people knew that drinking or eating contaminated food caused illness. In this category, such cases as abdominal pains, vomiting, diarrhoea and dysentery were placed. Sometimes, the food may not necessarily have been contaminated, but had been eaten when it had been improperly prepared. Thus, among Babukusu children were warned against eating certain termites, *kamaresi,* in a fresh state. If this happened, the children would suffer from severe trembling and vomiting.

Luyia therapeutic behaviour

The above discussion has shown that the Abaluyia believed that ill-health in people was brought about by a multiplicity of factors. Most of the illnesses could, however, be ascribed to what one may term as magico-religious forces. Nevertheless, the attribution of illness to multiple causes meant that therapy was equally sought in multiple systems and that the curative and preventive measures taken were both magical and empirical. These measures were based on accumulated knowledge and experience passed on from one generation to the other through the process of socialization.

The Abaluyia employed a number of methods to prevent misfortunes and/or illnesses. For example, it was believed that some diseases were contagious so that people suffering from such diseases had to be isolated from the rest of the community. Consequently, people suffering from such diseases as leprosy, epilepsy, bubonic plague, small pox, chicken pox and scabies were either isolated entirely, or sharing of communal facilities with them restricted. Even people suffering from common colds were not allowed to share drinking straws in beer parties with others. Lepers, especially, had to have their houses isolated from the village and contact with other people completely cut off. In the cases of people suffering from diarrhoea and dysentery, they were advised to bury their excreta and not to leave it on the surface.

Other preventive measures involved the use of charms and medicines, measures which were used to protect people from illnesses and misfortunes were ultimately ascribed to mystical forces. This protective magic was mainly employed against human agents of illness and misfortune (i.e. witches and sorcerers). Wagner (1970:182) argues that

> In warding off the evil practices of witches and sorcerers it offers protection at the same time against all diseases and misfortunes that are supposed to be wielded by them.

Protective magic was also used by people against bad intentions or actions of ordinary people, such as theft and intrigue. The common types of protective magic comprised objects that were generally known and hence could be collected by anybody. In addition, there were rare amulets and medicines which were purchased from diviners (*bafumu* or *avakumu*; sing. *omufumu* or *omukumu*) or from herbalists (known in olulogoli as *avali velunyasi;* sing. *omwali wolunyasi*). Since they were rare, they were considered to be more powerful than those that could simply be collected by anybody. People used these amulets and medicines to protect themselves from a variety of potential dangers and misfortunes one of which was to protect themselves from death-spell of a sorcerer. In another instance people used amulets to render themselves immune to the *kamaloko* of witches. Amulets were also used in the protection of children from the evil eye of a witch. Finally, people used amulets to protect themselves from being killed by lightning as well as the various dangers one might meet while travelling (Wagner, 1970).

Apart from these measures taken to avert disease or misfortune, the Abaluyia also had measures which aimed at counteracting mystical forces either by combating, neutralizing or destroying them once they became active. The first step in doing this was to discover the particular agent responsible for the illness, accident or other misfortune that had occurred. This diagnosis was done through the art of divination and once the cause of the illness or misfortune had been identified, the diviner also prescribed the appropriate measures which would serve to combat and neutralize the causes thus detected.

If the cause of the problem was shown to be due to ritual contamination (known in Lubukusu as *luswa*), violation of a taboo or breach of a rule of avoidance, the counter-measure was ritual purification. In most purification rites, a sheep was slaughtered and the victim was smeared with its stomach contents. Thereafter, the meat was ceremonially consumed by those present unless they were otherwise disqualified from eating the meat for one reason or another. Among Babukusu a strip of skin from the ceremonial sheep was put around the victim's right wrist to enhance the power of the lustration. On the other hand, if the problem had been brought about by a curse, then the first step in the treatment was to induce the person who uttered the curse to come and participate in the rite of lifting that curse. The basic feature of the lustration was the reconciliation of the person who uttered the curse with his or her victim. Once this had been done, the originator of the curse performed an act by which the original act that made the curse effective was undone or reversed.

In cases where the diagnosis revealed the cause of illness or misfortune to be witchcraft or sorcery, the victim had a number of possible counter-measures. One of them was to try and induce the sorcerer to undo or remove his magic through a ritual performance. Secondly, a certain rite could be performed to redirect the magic power back to its originator. Thirdly, one would try to locate the harmful substances and then render it harmless by destroying it. Fourth, the victim could employ an amulet which would then actively combat or neutralize the potency of the harmful substance; in this case, it was not necessary to see or get hold of the harmful substance itself. Finally, the victim could try to punish or even destroy the originator of the harmful magic. This could be done either by accusing the suspect to the clan elders, compelling him to submit to an ordeal or, if caught in the act, lynching him.

Of these five counteracting options, the commonest were detection and destruction of harmful magic, and the use of counter-magic. Among Babukusu, the detection of hidden substances was the work of an expert known as *omuliuli* (pl. *baliuli*) whose duty was to detect and remove these substances from wherever they had been hidden. (*Omuliuli* was equipped with the necessary magical power which enabled him to see charms which ordinary people could not see.) Once he had detected and removed the harmful substances, *kamaloko*, he directed that they be destroyed. The work of destroying these evil substances was left to the victim or close family members whereby the substances were taken to the nearest stream or river, burnt and the ashes thrown into the water to be carried away and thus render them harmless.

In the case of *bilasila*, the patient was taken to an expert known among the Avalogoli as *omulumiki*. This expert was always a woman and used the cupping-horn (*ekilumiki*) to remove the evil substances lodged in one's stomach. In this treatment, the expert first made two or three incisions and then placed the cupping horn, from the cow killed in a sacrifice, on the wound. She then proceeded to suck blood from the wound and in the process removed the evil substances. Sometimes, the expert did not use the cupping-horn, but simply massaged the patient's lower abdomen with an annointment made from ghee and medicines.

In some cases, the diviner revealed that the illness or misfortune was due to the spirit of dead relatives in which case the counteraction depended on whether the spirit was a benevolent or a malevolent one. In the former, a sacrificial rite was performed to appease the spirit responsible for the trouble. Among both Avalogoli and the Babukusu, the animal to be used had to be free from any blemishes (i.e. a lame animal, one with scars or one with faults on its skin, hoofs or teeth could not be used in such sacrifices). In addition, among the Babukusu, the animal had to be of the same sex as the spirit to whom it was offered.

On the other hand, persistently troublesome spirits were warded off and destroyed. Among the Avalogoli, the bones of a troublesome spirit were ritually dug up and then burned. However, among the Babukusu, *bisieno* were rendered harmless by trapping them and locking them in a pot. The pot was then taken to a stream and buried in the swampy soil of the valley bottom (Wagner, 1970).

Besides magico-religious experts, there were ordinary experts who dealt with different problems in society one of which was the bone-setter. When a person broke his limbs, he or she went for treatment to a bone-setter who first aligned the bones and then massaged the affected spot with fats. After this, he used bark strips from a certain pliable plant to ensure that the bones remained in the same position of alignment. There were also experts who dealt with teeth; broken teeth and those found to be very loose were extracted.

Women having problems with their pregnancies or deliveries turned to traditional birth attendants (TBAs) who were always women. If a pregnant woman had constant abdominal pains she went to a traditional birth attendant who would massage her stomach or give her medicines to cure her. TBAs also had the knowledge to tell whether the foetus was lying in its proper position and how old such a foetus was. These experts also assisted women who could not deliver normally and those experiencing problems with discharging the placenta.

Contemporary Traditional Medicine Among the Abaluyia

In the above discussion, I have attempted to describe the medical world as understood and practised by the Abaluyia in the pre-colonial period When British rule was established in Kenya, two accompanying institutions came into effect and these have had a fundamental impact on traditional medicine in the country — the Western school and the Christian church. The two institutions combined together to "civilize the natives", the essence of this "civilization" being to exert the virtues of the European civilization whilst at the same time condemning the "savageness" of African civilization. Consequently, many African institutions underwent radical changes during this period of colonization, one of which was traditional medicine. In this section, I wish to give a brief account of traditional medicine during the colonial and the post-colonial periods.

In the early years of colonization, both the government and the various Christian missions established modern health centres in what is now Western Province. For the first time, therefore, the Abaluyia had access to alternative health care systems. Those who sought treatment from these modern facilities marvelled at the way diseases were diagnosed and treated without recourse to mystical forces. However, for the vast majority of the people, European medical practices were treated with a lot of suspicion, and hence people continued to believe in and practise traditional medicine. In many cases, the victims combined visits to modern health centres with those to traditional healers, especially with regard to mental illness, infertility (in both men and women), male impotency, incessant ill-luck and accidents of whatever kind. Also, most people continued to observe food taboos as well as ritual prohibitions and other avoidances. Morever, most of the Abaluyia still believed in love magic and the power of the ancestral spirits over the living. Thus, amulets or talismans, were worn to enhance one's love from one's partner or to acquire new love, or to ward off danger emanating from mystical forces.

This was basically the picture of the Luyia health care practices at the time of independence and this picture has not changed much. Recent studies by Maithya (1992), Kiragu (n.d.) and Nyamwaya (1986) point to the fact that the Abaluyia still attribute illness and misfortunes to multiple causes as a result of which there are multiple therapeutic practices. In his study, Maithya (1992) discusses mental illness among Babukusu with regard to causation, perception and resources employed in the management of the problem. He discovered that among these people, the definitions of mental illness are varied, ranging from the disease of the head through abnormal behaviour to traditional illness. According to him, the aetiological concepts of mental illness include inter alia witchcraft, breaking of taboos, failure to offer sacrifices, accidents, organic illness (e.g. malaria) and chemical imbalance in the head (Maithya, 1992:172). The study also revealed that although therapies are multiple, traditional healers are the most preferred.

In his study among Abasamia, Nyamwaya (1986) discovered that these people recognize that poisoning, snake bites, 'mind' and physical degeneration cause illness, *obulwaye*. But when they try to explain the particularity of an illness, the Abasamia "resort to identifying things like witchcraft, violation of food and moral taboo and the evil eye, *obusura*, as "causes". Spirits, *ebikhieno*, especially *emisebe* (ancestor spirits), are also given as "causes" of certain conditions (Nyamwaya, 1986: 102). They classify diseases into those that are best treated at home and those best treated in modern health centres; those diseases whose causes appear to result from mystical forces are believed to be best treated at home and this category includes *ebikhieno*, measles, malnutrition, sorcery, infertility and madness. The Abasamia do not associate malnutrition with diet instead, they believe that this condition is due to either adultery or evil eye, *obusura* (see also K'Okul, 1991).

Therefore, many Abaluyia still believe that social, spiritual and psychological factors cause illness in people. To ensure that people do not suffer from illness due to these factors, most of them try to be in harmony with one another as well as with the living dead. In real life, however, it is not possible to maintain continuous harmony with other people or with the living dead. Now and again the living do certain things or fail to fulfill certain obligations and this annoys the ancestral spirits. To prevent negative consequences arising from this disharmony, the living perform certain rituals and ceremonies to appease the spirits. In order to determine the spirit which has been offended and what particular ritual or ceremony needs to be performed, or what course of action to take, people consult diviners, *bafumu* or *abalakusi* in some Luyia languages. These experts still exist in many parts of Buluyia and are consulted either openly or secretly, depending on the educational status, age and/or religious affiliations of the client. Old men and women with no or low formal education consult diviners openly whilst younger people with high educational levels tend to do so secretly, Those who ascribe to the various Christian denominations in the area also tend to consult diviners discretly.

If the cause of trouble is traced to a spirit who wants to eat, then a prescribed sacrifice is performed. As in the olden days, whatever animal is used in the sacrifice should be free from any blemishes. If, on the other hand, the cause is traced to *kamaloko*, the counteracting measures are either obtained from herbalists, *baliuli* or *avalumiki*.

However, contrary to the situation in the past, experts such as the bone-setter, traditional surgeon and the dentist are hardly used. If a person fractures his/her bones or suffers a dislocation, he/she will seek treatment in a modern health facility. The same applies to those who suffer from toothache or pneumonia. The traditional birth attendant is still very much in use; in fact, this expert has assumed a new significance as her expertise is being incorporated into the modern health delivery system whereby the TBAs spread throughout Buluyia have been trained in modern methods of hygiene to enable them perform their duties more efficiently. Whenever they are called upon to deliver babies, they carry with them first aid equipment as well as their certificates.

Today, traditional medicine has a new expert. This is a man or woman who combines the Bible and herbs to diagnose and treat a wide range of diseases. Mr.

Patrick Makokha (not his real name) is one such expert. He comes from Mumias Division of Kakamega District. Mr. Makokha uses the Bible to diagnose the problems of those who go to him to seek therapy. Once he has diagnosed the problem, he prescribes the course of action to be taken. If he prescribes herbal treatment, he goes ahead to dispense the necessary drug. If, on the other hand he diagnoses the problem as having been brought about by hidden charms, he tells the patient what type the charms are and then proceeds to pull them. This he does using the Bible and basket. The charms will be pulled from wherever they have been hidden and land in the basket. Mr. Makokha then takes the charms and hands them to the patient or whoever went to consult him on behalf of the patient with instructions regarding the destruction of the evil medicines. Finally, if it is the ancestors who want 'to eat', Mr. Makokha will prescribe the ritual or ceremony to be performed.

Conclusion

This chapter has attempted an overview of the Luyia traditional medical system. Examination of the system as it was before colonization as well as in the early part of the colonial period reveals that the agents and forces believed by the Abaluyia to cause diseases and misfortunes fall into five classes, namely the human factor, violations of taboos and ritual avoidances, ancestral spirits, environmental pollution and contaminated food. This means that these people believed that diseases and misfortunes were caused by a multiplicity of factors, a belief that meant that people sought treatment in a multiplicity of ways. Thus, the victims turned to diviners who identified the actual cause of the problem and then prescribed the course of action to be followed. Therapies included isolation of the victim (in cases of contagious disease), use of protective charms, appeasement of the living dead through sacrifices, use of herbs and the identification and destruction of harmful charms. In cases of biological diseases, herbs as well as other forms of treatment were offered.

In their traditional medical set-up, therefore, the Abaluyia had a number of healers. One of these was the herbalist, known in Olusamia as *omulesi* (pl. *abalesi*). The herbalist provided drugs that treated mystical diseases as well as ordinary diseases of a serious nature. Secondly, there was *omuliuli*, thirdly, divination was done by an expert the Abasamia referred to as *omulakusi* (pl. *obalakusi*). The fourth epert was known as *omulumiki* or *omulumikhi*, the person who physically removed harmful objects from the body of a patient. Fifthly, there were experts who treated fractures and dislocations, and those who removed aching or broken teeth. Finally, traditional birth attendants (TBAs) treated pregnant women and also helped them to deliver.

In general, one can state that despite the effects of colonialism and the attendant Western influences, the Luyia disease aetiologies have not changed dramatically. Recurrent illness or incessant misfortunes are still attributed to magico-religious factors. Choice of therapy in this case will normally fall on seeking measures that would counter the effects of what are perceived to be evil charms. However, in those areas where Christianity has been strongly rooted, most people no longer attribute illness or misfortunes to mystical factors. Such people will normally visit a modern health facility or buy over-the-counter proprietary drugs for self-medication when they fall sick. If modern medicines fail to cure the illness, the people are likely to first approach the evangelical healers found throughout Western Province for diagnosis and treatment of the illness. As a last resort, however, many Abaluyia will seek remedy from traditional healers. In most cases, people now combine visits to a modern health facility, traditional healers as well as to healers who combine the Bible and traditional medicine. In the end, the patient might not be in a position to know which of the healers actually cured his/her illness.

REFERENCES

Kiragu, F. K. "Medicine and Health". In *Bungoma District Socio-Cultural Profile: Draft Report* edited by G.S. Were. Nairobi: Institute of African Studies. pp. 143-153.

K'Okul, R. N. O. 1991. *Maternal and Child Health in Kenya; A Study of Poverty, Disease and Malnutrition in Samia.* Uppsala: Scandinavian Institute of African Studies.

Maithya, H. M. K. 1992. *The Awareness and Management of Mental Illness Among the Babukusu of Bungoma District.* M.A. Thesis, University of Nairobi.

Nyamwaya, D. 1986. "Medicine and Health." In *Kenya Socio-Cultural Profiles: Busia District* edited by G. S. Were. Nairobi: Ministry of Planning and National Development and Institute of African Studies. pp. 101-113.

Wagner, G. 1970. *The Bantu of Western Kenya, Vol. 1* London: Oxford University Press.

Chapter 11

KIKUYU TRADITIONAL MEDICINE*

Isaac Sindiga, Mary P. Kanunah
Eric M. Aseka, Gladys W. Kiriga,

This chapter first examines Kikuyu disease aetiologies and then discusses the role of the Kikuyu traditional medicineman (*mũndũ mũgo* pl. *andũ ago*) in society. Finally, it evaluates the contemporary status of Kikuyu traditional medicine.

Background

The Bantu-speaking Kikuyu are the largest single ethnic group in Kenya making up 21 per cent of the country's population (Kenya, 1994: 6-2). They numbered over four million in the 1989 population census. They occupy five districts of Central Province, namely Kiambu, Nyeri, Nyandarua, Thika and Murang'a and are heavily represented in the former White Highlands especially in the Rift Valley Province. They are also widely scattered in many areas of the country.

Kikuyu settlement in central Kenya goes back to more than four centuries. Murang'a District is considered to be their ancestral and spiritual home (Muriuki, 1976;1974).

Much has been written about the Kikuyu—their history and society (Muriuki, 1974) and their life and customs (Leakey, 1977; Kenyatta 1978; Gathigira, 1952). We therefore have relied on the available anthropological literature to piece together this sketch about Kikuyu traditional medicine.

Kikuyu Disease Aetiologies

Kikuyu traditional medicine is closely linked with the cosmological beliefs of the

* Two separate chapter drafts on this subject were independently prepared, one by Eric Aseka and Gladys Kiriga, and another by Isaac Sindiga and Mary Kanunah. The latter co-authors put this chapter together from the two submissions.

people. In particular, medicine is intertwined with religion and magical practices (Kenyatta, 1978). In fact, so complex is the web of interaction between magical and medical practices that Kenyatta (1978) discusses them together and does not appear to differentiate them.

The Kikuyu appear to have very clear ideas as to what causes disease (*mũrimũ*). This provides the basis for therapy and the management of a given problem. Table 1.1 provides a classification of the causes of ill health as put forward by Leakey (1977: 836-936). This categorization represents a descriptive effort which illuminates the nature rather than the causes of disease and ill health among the precolonial and colonial Kikuyu. However, Kikuyu disease aetiologies can be distilled into at least four categories; natural, supernatural, and human-induced causes, and breaching taboos.

As noted in Chapter 2, natural diseases are those that are thought to emanate from environmental conditions. Among the traditional Kikuyu, such were recognised because they could be cured using herbal treatments (Kenyatta, 1978:20). Virtually all Kikuyu elders had some knowledge of the herbal remedies for various conditions (Leakey, 1977:1145) so that a sick family member was at first given medicine at home, and only when he failed to respond to such medication was he taken to a "professional" healer (Leakey, 1977; cf. the Maasai case detailed in Chapter 8).

The Kikuyu also believed that diseases could be caused by a supernatural power or ancestral spirits, which beliefs hold that the spirits of the dead can be pleased or displeased by the behaviour of a person, family or even an age-group. According to Kenyatta (1978:267) there are at least four categories of spirits as follows:

1. Spirits of the father or mother (*ngoma cia aciari*)
2. Clan spirits (*ngoma cia mũhĩrĩga*)
3. Age-group spirits (*ngoma cia riika*); and
4. Gikuyu spirits (*ngoma cia rũrĩrĩ*)

Ngoma cia aciari usually communicate directly with living children to offer advice or to complain about wrong-doing. *Ngoma cia mũhĩrĩga* are responsible for watching over the general welfare and prosperity of the clan. On the other hand, *ngoma cia riika* are concerned with the activities of particular age-groups. Finally, there appears to be *ngoma cia rũrĩrĩ* which watch over the welfare of the entire Kikuyu tribe (Kenyatta, 1978).

The various ancestral spirits were believed to live in the bushes around homesteads. Sometimes they would become angry and launch a massive attack on the people across a large area. Such spirits were said to be carried by the wind from one homestead to another and were responsible for epidemic disease

Table 11.1: Causes of ill health among the pre-colonial Kikuyu

Category/Cause	Disease	Kikuyu name
1. Infectious epidemic diseases		
	— smallpox	*mũtũngũ*
	— chicken-pox	*mũthandũkũ*
	— measles	*mũthũũkũ* or *gĩthũ*
	— mumps	*mũngai*
2. Infectious, non-epidemic diseases		
	— yaws	*mũcarĩ*
	— gonorrhoea	*gatego/gĩcũnũnũ*
	— bilharzia	*mũthĩorĩ*
3. Illness due to natural causes*		
	— dysentery	*gatema*
	— diarrhoea	*rũharo*
	— tapeworms	ndangũrũ
	— constipation	*Kũũmĩrũo nĩ nda*
	— rheumatism	*mahĩndĩ*
	— fever and colds	*kĩhuti*
	— severe chest cold	*rũhayo*
	— cough	*gũkorora*
	— eye infection	*kũrũara maitho*
	— suppurating ear	*njiika*
	— toothache	*kũrĩo nĩ igego*
	— boils	*mahũha*
	— nose bleeding	*nũnũho*
	— warts	*mbatata*
	— scabies	*ũhere*
	— itching	*mwĩthũa*
	— elephantiasis	*rũbai/matende*
	— leprosy	*mangũ*
	— sores	*ironda*
	— burns	*mahĩa*
	— whitlows	thita
	— swollen testicles	*iganĩ*
	— distended stomach	*ihu ria mũthũthũma*
	— heartburn	*kĩrũngũrĩra*
	— hiccups	*kĩegetha*
	— sciatic nerve	*inangethũ*
	— liver pain	*gũcũnwo nĩ ini*
	— gall sickness	*ndigana*
	— cuts, wounds	*gũtemwo, ironda*
	— snake bite	*kũrũmwo nĩ nyoka.*
4. Sickness caused by supernatural powers and/or ancestral spirits**		
5. Sickness caused by witchcraft		*ũrogi*
6. Sickness caused by breaching taboos		*mĩgiro*

* recognized because they can be cured using herbs (Kenyatta, 1978:290).

** Sudden attack by unknown disease or failure to obtain cure of known condition after using herbal remedies.

SOURCES: *The Southern Kikuyu Before 1903* by L.S.B. Leakey (1977) pp. 383-936, and *Facing Mount Kenya* by J. Kenyatta (1978), p. 290.

outbreaks (Kenyatta, 1978). These spirits could also maintain diseases in endemic form within an area.

During the precolonial and colonial periods, infectious epidemic diseases, including smallpox, chickenpox, measles and mumps, wreaked havoc in Kikuyuland. Although they occurred periodically, they could cause suffering across wide areas and among many people. Once an epidemic broke out, Kikuyu elders got together to determine the cause of the affliction and how to manage it; usually, they would consult specialist seers or diviners on the actual cause of the misfortune and how the people could be relieved.

According to Leakey (1977), smallpox (*mũtũngũ*) and chickenpox *(mũthandũkũ)* were understood to derive from the evil spirits in the land. Victims of the former were abandoned in the bush in a temporary shelter from where they were monitored and nursed in the hope that they would recover. In addition to isolating them, the Kikuyu developed a method of vaccination, whereby those who had recovered from a previous attack of the disease were made to play the role of vaccinators. Recovering patients were made to give their serum through the pricking of the pustules and squeezing the pus onto a leaf. This was rubbed onto cuts in the skins of the newly infected. They merely conceived the transfer process in terms of transporting worn out and weary spirits and that is why a recovered patient had to undergo a process of purification before being accepted into the society once more. The purification process entailed rubbing his whole body with undigested stomach contents (*taatha*) of a rum (Leakey, 1977:889-891).

Unlike smallpox, those suffering from chickenpox were not kept in seclusion. However, it was believed that chickenpox brought smallpox. Thus the appearance of chickenpox led to the employment of quick measures to ceremonially chase away evil spirits from Kikuyuland (Leakey, 1977:891-892). Another disease was measles (*gĩthũkũ*). When it broke out, the Kikuyu resorted to magical means to curb its spread. A concoction from red ochre and earth from a mole-hill mixed with sugar-cane beer was applied on the rashes. Another application was the rubbing of leaves of a plant called *terere* (*Amaranthus hybridus*) over the patient's whole body so that the plant juice could penetrate the skin (Leakey, 1977:892-893).

An outbreak of mumps (*mũngai*) also elicited a concerted effort to drive the evil spirits away from the land. Whereas, among the Luyia of Western Kenya, the infected person danced around a tree called *omurembe (Erythrina abyssinica)* with a bundle of firewood while chanting that the mumps should remain there after which he was supposed to bolt from the spot without looking back, the Kikuyu did something very close to this. The victim "stood infront of a *mũtũndũ* tree *(Croton onacrostachyus)* and addressed it as though it was a human being" by stating "***mũtũndũ iyũkia mũngai waku***" (*mũtũndũ* tree, take your mumps) (Leakey, 1977: 893-894). This was a typical case of psychotherapy.

This association of health problems with the supernatural showed that Africans are "ethico-religious" and catastrophies are seen as manifestations of anger of the supreme being. Alternatively, such phenomena were cause by evil forces (Onwuanibe, 1978:1); that is, sickness of whatever kind is attributable to human and supernatural causation. In determining the people's perception of the seriousness of diseases, ethico-religious considerations were important variables. They also played a significant role in the medical practitioner's assessment of the relative efficacy of traditional alternatives in the control and management of such diseases (Thomas, 1970:173).

Among the infectious and non-epidemic maladies that the pre-colonial Kikuyu grappled with were yaws *(mũcarĩ)*, gonorrhoea and bilharzia, which were collectively termed *mũthiori*. Yaws was a dreaded disease, curable only when diagnosed and managed immediately after an attack. Those afflicted were shunned and avoided but there were medicinemen with the expertise of immunizing people in the community against yaws. The common treatment involved chopping up and boiling little chunks of the branches of the *mũteta* tree (*Strychnos henningsii*). Hot water infused with the juices of the tree then mixed with honey constituted herbal medicine often used in its treatment. Another treatment involved extraction of fluid from a plant called *mũtũkia* and boiling it after which the liquid was "applied to all open sores" Leakey, 1977:894-895).

Mũthiori victims were also given herbal medicine. Roots of various plants, including sorghum and banana plants, were gathered and boiled together for a given period. Thereafter "the water was then strained off and mixed with fresh cow's milk, and sometimes with a little mutton fat" (Leakey, 1977:895). After storage in a gourd for three days, the patient then drunk a hornful of the concoction three times a day and was expected to obtain relief in two to five days. Societal norms forbade such victims from indulging in sexual intercourse and sharing a bed (Leakey, 1977:895).

Ill health could also be human-induced. The major culprits here were *arogi* (witches). Among the Kikuyu, witchcraft (*ũrogi*) involved magical use of herbs for destructive reasons (Kenyatta, 1978). These herbs could be used to poison the victims thereby causing sickness and perhaps death. Thus, there were charms used to destroy friendship (*mũnuunga* or *rũruto*) and those used for protection against witchcraft (*gĩthiitũ*). Traditionally, the majority of the Kikuyu carried a charm for protection against all dangers (Kenyatta, 1978).

Sorcerers and witches were most hated in Kikuyu society. Once found out, they were forced to eat their poison after which they were killed. This was done either by throwing them down a steep slope in a giant beehive, or by burying them alive (Thairu, 1975:85).

Finally, the Kikuyu believed that sickness could be caused by breaking tribal laws and customs governing social relationships. Such included sexual impropriety among married people (Leakey, 1977:933). If the individual involved did not repent, he or she could pay the ultimate price of death or attract supernatural misfortune to self and/or family.

Manpower in Kikuyu Traditional Medicine

A Kikuyu medicineman *(mũndũ mũgo)* was a most respected person within the community (Thairu, 1975:85; Kenyatta, 1978; Leakey, 1977). Normally, only men could become *andũ ago*. Occasionally, however, a woman became *nyitwo nĩ ũgo*, that is, possessed by magic thereby becoming a famous prophetess, seer or healer (Leakey, 1977:1152). However, as shall be shown below, each medicineman had to undergo an elaborate initiation ceremony in order to become recognised as a healer. A woman healer did not participate in the all-important initiation ceremony and did not possess a divining gourd. For the women healers,

> Their prestige and power was based upon their ability to prophesy accurately, and their reputation of being in such close contact with the deity as to receive messages directly from Him (sic) (Leakey, 1977:1152).

A Kikuyu medicineman (*mũndũ mũgo*) is also known by several other terms none of which fully conveys the required meaning; healer, diviner, seer, magician and "witchdoctor". Leakey, (1977) noted that Kikuyu traditional medical practice was a serious and demanding vocation for only the chosen ones who, in addition, had to go through training and initiation.

An individual was specifically called upon to join the profession of *ũgo*. This calling was demonstrated by a person serving as an apprentice to his kin, for example, a son learning the father's vocation or a person serving on apprenticeship with a *mũndũ mũgo*. Sometimes, a child was born clutching a diviner's counter (*mbũgũ*) (i.e. a smooth white pebble) in his fist (Leakey, 1977:1224). Such a child was earmarked to become a *mũndũ mũgo* when he grew older. In other instances, the calling came in late childhood or adulthood. This would usually be manifested by lengthy illness, with such symptoms as dreams, fits, hallucinations, aberrant behaviour or vision difficulties as well as a series of misfortunes befalling a person, including death of children and failure to prosper (Leakey, 1977:1123; Good, Kimani and Lawry, 1980:88). In whatever category the calling fell, it was believed that the deity wanted the individual to be a *mũndũ mũgo*. As such, *andũ ago* had a very special relationship with God (*Ngai*). Indeed, one could not practise successfully without God's assistance (Leakey, 1977: 1124). Part of the reverence that *andũ ago* secured in traditional society derived from their perceived close relationship with *Ngai*.

As already noted, traditional medical practitioners were both generalists and specialists; however, a healer could combine several specialities (Thairu, 1975:85). The specializations included divination, identifying witches and sorcerers, prophecy, herbalism, anti-witchcraft and purification, infertility among women, mental illness, and conjuring and hypnosis (psychiatry) (Good, Kimani and Lawry, 1980:88; Thairu, 1975:85). Another specialization in traditional medicine was the treatment of fractures, suturing wounds and conducting certain operations (Thairu, 1985). *Andũ ago* understood wound infection and asepsis and took appropriate steps to handle the problems. The duties of the medicinemen varied as well; they ranged from healing, blessing and purifying the defiled, to appeasing ancestral spirits. In addition, they worked as counsellors and ritual experts (Thairu, 1975:85; Kenyatta, 1978:291).

General practitioners conducted purification rites and ceremonies in normal social life. They cured diseases referred to them by elders and prepared and administered minor charms to prevent illness and bring good fortune while on safari. According to Leakey, (1977:146), not all *andũ ago* could divine — only about 10 per cent of them specialized in *ũragũri* (divination and prophecy). In fact, general practitioners were excluded from certain categories of divination, which were instead handled by specialists. Thus, in cases of severe drought, crop failure or warriors preparing for a battle with the Maasai, specialist diviners (who were seen as prophets with supernatural power), were consulted (Leakey1977: 1150-1151).

Initiation of a mũndũ mũgo

Notwithstanding how a *mũndũ mũgo* was called into the healing profession, he could not start to practise and to charge fees until he was "licensed". Such licensing took the form of initiation in an elaborate and expensive ceremony lasting three days. The initiation ceremony was called *gũkũnũra mũgo*— to uncover the *mũgo* (Leakey 1977:1124). This ceremony has been discussed in detail by Leakey (1977) for the Kikuyu of Kiambu; Good, Kimani and Lawry (1980) for the Kikuyu of Murang'a; and Gathigira (1952) for the Kikuyu of the northern side or Nyeri. The *gũkũnũra mũndũ mũgo* ceremony was led by an experienced traditional healer who then became the mentor of the newly admitted man. Admission into the practice was symbolized by possession of divining gourds and magic powers which were necessary in the work of *mũndũ mũgo*. Also, every qualified *mũndũ mũgo* carried a charm called *gĩthitũ kĩrĩa kĩnene* (Leakey 1977:1142).

Ethics in traditional medical practice

In discussing training and specializations in traditional medical practice, Leakey (1977) noted that it compared favourably to the standards of Western medicine. Leakey writes:

> . . . the profession was one that could not be entered into light-heartedly, and moreover, one at which it was by no means easy to be successful. In fact, quite a number of those who were initiated into the profession failed to make a success of it and ceased to practice.

A *mũndũ mũgo* was enjoined to keep the confidentiality of the health and social problems of his clients. A traditional healer who divulged such information was severely reprimanded by colleagues or "would be so cursed by them that he would not recover" (Leakey 1977: 1121). Because of this requirement, clients would be expected to be quite open about their problems when making consultations with *andũ ago*.

Kikuyu medicinemen knew their limitations as well. They usually admitted their inability to offer therapy to hopeless cases. In such instances, a *mũndũ mũgo* would declare to his assistants and others: "*Kũnja mbũri na rũa, mũndũ nĩ witũ na Ngai*" (Fold the ceremonial goat meat with the goatskin and let's get the hell out of here. The life of this sick man now lies between me and God!)" (Thairu, 1975: 86). Similarly, a general practitioner would make referrals of cases he could not handle to specialist *andũ ago*.

Contemporary Kikuyu Traditional Medicine

With the advent of colonialism in Kikuyuland early in the 20th century, a number of actions were taken to discourage certain aspects of African culture including traditional medicine. The colonial administration set up modern health facilities begrudgingly (Sindiga, 1990). In the meantime, Christian churches competed to carve out areas of influence — the Church of Scotland Mission, the Roman Catholic Church and Church Missionary Society were some of the earliest to establish themselves in Kikuyuland. These groups created modern health facilities in their areas of operation.

The new administrators as well as the preachers in the midst of the Kikuyu pressed for the abandonment of certain cultural practices, among them traditional medicine. Government policy called for the setting up of government hospitals and rendering assistance to the ones run by missionaries (Sindiga, 1990:134). But as efforts in the expansion of modern medicine were gaining momentum, some legislative actions were taken to stifle traditional medicine. Such included the Witchcraft Act of 1925 (revised in 1962) which aimed at protecting Kenyans from fear or intimidation by "witchdoctors" (Sindiga, 1990:138; see also Chapter 3). Despite this Act, people who had no faith in modern medicine continued to utilize traditional medicine. In addition, the Kikuyu discovered that the new medicine could not effectively address their medico-social problems. This was especially so for diseases which required some form of ritual performance and purification to exorcise spirits.

Given the negative tag which had been given to traditional medical practice, many people resorted to concealing their visits to traditional medical practitioners in order to avoid creating conflict with either their fellow Christians, or the colonial administration. The situation necessitated visiting distant areas/places for this form of medical care as part of concealment. One such place was Ukambani whereby some people utilized Kamba herbalists and medico-religious specialists or specialists with powers of divination to guard against misfortune. Even the Akamba themselves were caught up in this conflict of interest over medical care. They resorted to traditional alternatives where modern medicine was ineffective (Thomas, 1970).

The colonial stereotypes about traditional medicine and the influence of missionary admonitions have yet to be overcome in contemporary Kikuyu society; they carry forth to the present time. Kikuyu traditional medicine exhibits a general lack of co-ordination. The *andũ ago* are scattered in the countryside. Good and his colleagues observed rural traditional medicine among the Kikuyu to be in a process of decay, and the "mainly elderly practitioners are perhaps the last generation of rural *andũ ago*" (Good, Kimani and Lawry, 1980:89).

Kikuyu Christians are against traditional medicine. Perhaps we should note that Kikuyuland has undergone profound socio-economic changes over the past 100 years and as noted above, culture has not been spared. The significance of the initiation of traditional healers, *gũkunũra mũndũ mũgo* is diminishing. In fact,

> An enterprising, prospective practitioner of traditional medicine need not obtain the formal validation required of his ancestors if he can (1) demonstrate an acquaintance with herbs and magic perhaps through an informal apprenticeship with an elder *mũndũ mũgo* and (2) easily build rapport with and satisfy many of the psychotherapeutic needs of his clients (Good, Kimani and Lawry, 1980:115).

In general, the role of the *mũndũ mũgo* has been minimized with the emergence of complex social relations characterized by intense contacts and cosmopolitan value formation. The place of *mũndũ mũgo* has been replaced by quasi-modern traditional practitioners who have attempted to marry traditional and modern methods. Some of these are educated herbal practitioners who are increasingly using modern equipment to diagnose sickness but give herbal dispensations. Such is the case with Jack Githae (See Chapter 5).

Some of the clinics belonging to these practitioners are equipped with modern medical paraphernalia whose cost is compensated by the upward adjustment of their charges. However, compared to fees charged at official health facilities, most of them are relatively cheap. This is because their medicine is made from locally available herbs, roots, leaves, stems and tree barks which may be boiled, ground to powder form or otherwise. Their medicine preparation is governed by a highly secretive resolve that is perhaps meant to minimize the number of competitors.

Other traditional practitioners still operating secretly among the Kikuyu are circumcision surgeons (for both boys and girls) and traditional birth attendants (TBAs). There are also those herbalists who are barely literate and mainly operate or practice in the countryside. The majority of the practitioners in this category combine their roles as herbalists with other activities like farming.

The institution of magic practitioners and other divinational experts is increasingly becoming more and more camouflaged. As quasi-modern herbal practitioners emerge and publicize their abilities through the media and personal contacts, the divinational experts have gone into hiding and the art may die.

We detect an adaptive dimension in traditional medicine. Kikuyu herbal practitioners are increasingly adapting themselves to social changes in society and are performing their roles in accordance with the needs of the communities which constitute their clientele (Githagui, 1985:70; Good, Kimani and Lawry, 1980). Indeed patients from different ethnic backgrounds in the country seek their services. These include men and women of varying ages and both literate and non-literate. Also, they comprise the rich and the poor.

It appears that increased urbanization is contributing to the migration of traditional healers into urban centres where they are setting up their practices on a commercial basis (Good, Kimani and Lawry, 1980). The shortage of drugs in health facilities and the lack of such facilities in some areas in the country is boosting the growth in their clientele. The presence of "difficult diseases", where patients have not responded positively to modern medicine over a long period of time, is yet another factor explaining the persistence of herbal practice. Indeed practitioners clearly point out that the bulk of the patients they treat will have tried modern medicine without success. Most of them carry along the documentation of their medical history to the herbalist.

Conclusion

Kikuyu traditional medicine is in a state of change. It persists in a subdued manner in the rural areas of Kikuyuland. This is because "most people, regardless of their background or station in life, continue to respect and even fear the potential power of *andũ ago* (Good, Kimani and Lawry, 1980:115). However, a modified form of traditional medicine is booming in urban places. This surely suggests continued patronage.

REFERENCES

Gathigira, S.K. 1952. *Mũkarĩre ya Agĩkũyũ*. London: Sheldon Press.

Githagui, N. 1985. *Traditional Healing Practices in Kenya: A Story of Four Kenyan Communities.* Nairobi: AMREF.

Good, C. M., V. Kimani and J. M. Lawry. 1980. "*Gũkunũra Mũndũ Mũgo*: The initiation of a Medicineman." *Anthropos* Vol. 75:87-116.

Kenya, Government of. 1994. *Kenya Population Census 1989 Volume 1.* Nairobi: Government Printer.

Kenyatta, J. 1978. *Facing Mount Kenya.* Nairobi: Heinemann Educational Books.

Leakey, L. S. B. 1977. *The Southern Kikuyu Before 1903 Vols I, II and III.* London: Academic Press.

Muriuki, G. 1974. *A History of the Kikuyu 1500-1900.* Nairobi: Oxford.

________. 1976. "The Kikuyu in the Pre-Colonial Period." In *Kenya Before 1900: Eight Regional Studies* edited by B.A. Ogot. Nairobi: East African Publishing House. pp. 106-138.

Onwuanibe, B.C. 1978. "The Philosophy of African Medical Practice." Paper presented at the 21st Annual Meetings of the African Studies Association, Baltimore, Maryland, November, 1-4.

Sindiga, I. 1990. "Health and Disease". In *Themes in Kenya History* edited by W. R. Ochieng. Nairobi: Heinemann. pp. 133-144.

Thairu, K. 1975. *The African Civilization.* Nairobi: East African Literature Bureau.

Thomas, A. E. 1970. *Adaptation to Modern Medicine in Lowland Machakos. Kenya: A Controlled Comparison of Two Kamba Communities.* Ph. D Dissertation, Stanford University.

Chapter 12

THE ROLE OF TRADITIONAL MEDICINE IN A RURAL ENVIRONMENT

S. R. Baquar

Introduction

Traditional herbal medicines play a vital role towards the well-being and development of the rural population in Kenya. Herbal therapy, though still an unwritten science, is well established in the cultures and traditions and has become a way of life of almost 80 per cent of the people in Africa. Local herbs have been used since time immemorial, in time of war as well as in time of peace because plants have both healing and killing properties, depending on the knowledge of their dosage and synergistic action. And this is well known to traditional medicinemen whose experience in dealing with such herbs should not be underestimated or considered inferior in any way to the Western method of treatment.

It has been noted that many diseases which could not be cured by the allopathic or other systems of treatment have been cured by traditional medicine. The social acceptance of traditional medicine by a majority of people is based on various factors, the primary ones being its accessibility and its cheap cost of healing. Local herbs have great potential of healing and many of them have found utility in foreign markets and are exploited commercially. Many natural drugs, extracted from the plants, can be duplicated synthetically in the laboratories which may be more reliable in terms of the known active principles. However, the side-effects of many purified synthetic chemical drugs may be alarming as compared to the natural drugs. Symptoms such as dizziness, blurred vision, palpitation or rashes caused by some of the chemical drugs are well known and have been experienced by many of us. It is for this reason that the traditional medicines are still considered safe in many ways.

A thorough and systematic survey, collection, identification and proper documentation of such medicinal herbs, with a view to building a germplasm collection, is of prime importance to Kenya. The local medicinemen could be taken into confidence and lured to reveal their healing magic for the benefit of the community at large. Every year, a large quantity of drugs is imported, which import requires a significant proportion of the hard earned foreign exchange at the cost of many other important items. This financial constraint could be reduced and money diverted towards more pressing needs if local drug industries are encouraged and vitalized for the exploitation of local herbs.

Historical Perspective

The history of herbal medicine is rather old and dates back to when the early man became conscious of his surroundings. Cultural man is said to have been on earth for some two or three million years and throughout the greater part of the period, he has struggled for his existence as a hunter-gatherer. Thousands of years of experience, by trial and error must have taught him to distinguish between useful and harmful plants with their properties as healing agents dawning on him much later. To become conscious of their utility and applicability as medicinal herbs, must have taken him another large portion of his existence (Baquar, 1991).

The earliest record of human civilization and culture of China, Egypt, Assyria and Indus Valley reveals that the elders and wisemen of those times used herbal medicines to treat various diseases. Information regarding these medicinal herbs is available in the old literature, folklore, mythological stories, epic poems, medicinal treatises and thousands — years old manuscripts, palm leaves and copper plates and other records on these cultures which are preserved even today. The excavation of Shanidar cave in Iraq in 1963 revealed the grave of the Neanderthal man buried sixty thousand years ago along with many flowers of his time. The plants found in the grave were later identified through palynological studies to be having various medicinal properties such as diuretic, emetic astringent, stimulant and pain reliever (Lehane, 1977).

Thousands of years before the development of farming or any other kind of civilization nomadic and primitive people had a considerable knowledge of plant medicine. The earliest references to the use of medicinal herbs as a cure for diseases is found in the manuscript of "Eber Papyrus" in about 16th century B.C. which recorded the use of poppy (*Papaver somnifera*), castor oil (*Ricinus communis*), squills (*Urginea* sp.) and aloes (Aloe sp.). Theophrastus (370-287 BC), an outstanding Greek naturalist, in his "Enquiry into Plants" mentions

> he who would obtain peony (*Paeonia* sp.) roots was advised to dig it up at night because if he did the deed in daytime, and was observed by wood pickers he risked the loss of his eye-sight.

He described 500 plants mostly cultivated. Pliny the Elder (23-79 A.D.), a Roman naturalist and philosopher, describes 1000 plants with their medicinal properties, anatomy and horticultural practices in his book, *Historia Naturalis*. Dioscorides (1st century A.D.), a military physician during the reign of Nero (the harsh Emperor of Rome) wrote "De Material Medica", describing 600 plant species of medicinal value from the Mediterranean region. Another manuscript, the *Anicia Juliana Codex*, was prepared for the daughter of Byzantine Emperor about 512 A.D. from material originally compiled by Dioscorides. It contains coloured illustrations of plants and is still in existence.

For a long time, medicinal plants have been the subject of study and their value and method of treatment has hardly changed since those mentioned in the Ayurvedic and Greeko-Arab systems and the Allopathaic and the Homeopathic literature. Men have used the herbs quite intuitively for food as well as for bodily ailments and thus maintained their health in perfect condition throughout their long life. Long ago it was believed that each plant was created for the benefit of man and a close observation of these plants would reveal some sign or "signature" indicating its proper use. Plants with some parts resembling the lobes of a liver were supposed to be useful for the remedy of liver ailment, while those having resemblance to the heart, say cordate leaves of various plants, would be used against heart diseases. The reddish juice of pomegranate was considered to be good for blood diseases. Plants with trailing or winding stem in the grass, would help to cure the snake bite. The flowers of *Aristolochia* sp., curled up like an unborn baby, would help in easing the child birth and so on.

Many plants have been credited with supernatural powers and the knowledge of such plants was considered prestigious and it brought the physician closer to the rulers of the time. Witchdoctors, shamans and priests owed their standing to plants and to the peculiar rites and beliefs associated with gathering and processing them (Lehane, 1977). Mandrake, for example, is a poisonous plant with white or purple flowers and large yellow fruits having emetic and narcotic properties. Its roots, once thought to resemble human form and to shriek when plucked, were used as charm and carried by women of Eastern Europe as a charm against sterility. In Assyria mandrake was used to ward off plague and to induce sleep, relieve pain, cure baldness and as an aphrodisiac. The plant *Valeriana officinalia* is known as All-heal and its medicinal properties are endless.

Importance of Traditional Herbal Medicine

Indigenous medicinal herbs form an important component of the natural wealth of any country and have played a vital role towards the welfare of rural environment since the advent of history. In most of the developing countries, however, the information on plant resources is usually scattered and needs collection, revision and updating.

Traditional medicine is practised throughout the world, especially in the rural areas of Asia, Latin America and Africa. The rural population of a country is more disposed to traditional ways of treatment because of its easy availability and cheaper cost. Many remote areas in this region are beyond easy access using proper roads and communication lines both of which are prerequisites for access to modern medical care. Kenya, with a population of about 25 million people and an annual growth rate of 3.8 percent has a ratio of 1:1000 and 1:70,000 physicians in urban and rural areas respectively (Koinange, 1982).

In a situational analysis Koinange reports that "our nation's health resources, both public and private, are disproportionately allocated to our urban as compared to non-urban areas". He further says that "census data reveals nearly 87% of our population resides in rural areas, yet nearly 80% of our health resources are concentrated in our major cities of Nairobi and Mombasa". It is, therefore, understandable that the rural population is more dependent upon and contented with the traditional system of medicine.

Plants have provided man with a storehouse of various drugs where he can search for medicines for practically all ailments. The big pharmaceutical companies are in pursuit of drugs that are reputed for their therapeutic values with their representatives vigorously looking for information on such drugs. This information, however, has been stored in the minds of the rural medicinemen for generations. (It is no wonder that if the history of some of the important modern lifesaving drugs were to be traced it may lead us to the backyard of a rural medicineman). Traditional medicine is still an unwritten science; information, on the healing properties of certain medicinal herbs is kept secret by the traditional healers and passed on, from generation to generation, within families only. With few exceptions, these medicinemen or *waganga* (Swahili) tend to conceal such information and are very reluctant to part with their healing magic.

The use of medicinal herbs is, at times, accompanied by various rituals, including the chanting of traditional songs, wearing of amulets, burning of incense and witchcraft. This is probably because in the early days disease was believed to be connected with the attack of evil spirits and therefore witchcraft and traditional rituals were considered to be an antidote for the influence of evil spirits and alteration of fortune in one's favour. All these customs are still in practice in many parts of the world.

Some Herbal Drugs of Universal Importance

Some of the most important drugs have been extracted from plants and are fully exploited commercially. These drugs include: morphine from poppy (opium) plant (*Papaver somnifera*), cocaine from coca plant (*Erythroxylum coca*), strychnine from *Strychnos nux-vomica,* digitalin from foxglove (*Digitalis purpurea*), atropine from deadly nightshade (*Atropa belladona*), cannabis from bhang plant (*Cannabis sativa*), hyoscyamin from henbane (*Hyoscyamus niger*), aconitine from *Aconitum* sp., quinine from cinchona trees (*Cinchona officianalis, C. ledgeriana, C. cordifolia*), mandrogorine from mandarek (*Mandrax officinarum*) and ergotamine, ergometrine and ergotoxin from ergot (*Clavisceps purpurea*).

The discovery of *Penicillin,* derived from *Penicillium*, a common fungus and chloromycetin from a common actinomycetes belonging to a group of lower plants, was almost neglected for quite some time before its rediscovery and has now revolutionized the world and opened new vistas in the modern antibiotics.

The following herbal drugs have attained universal acclamation and are used commercially:

Aconitum napellus (Ranunclulaceae) is a deadly poisonous herb which contains the alkaloid aconitine. It acts on the central nervous system and is therefore used as a pain reliever as well as in heart complaints. The tincture can be applied externally in rheumatic and other pains. The plant is used as a tonic, febrifuge, antiperiodic and sedative. It is a highly poisonous drug.

Helleborus niger (Solanaceae) has a glycoside and is used as diuretic or purgative. The decoction is applied as poultice to children having lice. The plant is highly poisonous and even the external application may be dangerous.

Hyoscyamus niger (Solanaceae). The leaves of henbane (*Hyoscyamus niger*) contain active alkaloid and its oil is used externally as a balm to cure pain. The leaves are used as sedative, narcotic and in the treatment of asthma and whooping cough. They are smoked to treat toothache. Its chemical constituents are similar to those of deadly nightshade (*Atropa belladona*).

Atropa belladona (Solanaceae). The alkaloid atropine, extracted from *Atropa belladona* is an important component of the eye surgery to dilate the pupil. All parts of the plant are narcotic and poisonous. If taken internally, it can increase the rate of heartbeat. It is also used to prevent spasm of the stomach and for inhibiting the production of saliva and mucus in the lungs. In moderate quantity belladona can induce hallucination and deep sleep.

Datura stramonium (Solanaceae). This plant is found throughout tropical and subtropical regions. The alkaloid, daturine, extracted from this plant has symptoms similar to belladona. The decoction is inhaled in asthma but it has been found to aggravate bronchitis.

Digitalis purpurea (Scrophulariaceae). The plant is found in temperate regions. Leaf decoction of this herb is used to increase the flow of urine. Its main effect is on heartbeat which slows down, increasing its efficiency and reducing congestion in the veins.

Rauwolfia serpentina (Apocyanaceae). The plant is found in India, Bangladesh and Indonesia and was known to Ayurvedic physicians in ancient India (nearly 3000 years ago). Several alkoloids have been extracted from roots as serpentine, serpentinine, reserpine, rauwolfine and serpajmaline which act as a tranquilizer, for reducing blood pressure and for slowing the heartbeat. Patients of mental illness, insomnia and high blood pressure respond very well to this drug.

Strychnos nux-vomica (Loganiaceae). In South East Asia this tree has been used as medicine for centuries. The seed contains the alkaloid strychnine and brucine which stimulate the nervous system and increase secretion of gastric juices, sharpens appetite and promote digestion. It increases mental alertness, improves vision, and is effective in the treatment of paralysis. It is also considered as tonic, laxative and prophylactic against snake–bite and cholera. Its poison was used on criminals as it causes cramps, convulsion and an intense feeling of fear.

Ephedra sp. (Ephedraceae). Ephedras are leafless woody shrubs scattered all over the world. A decoction of the stem and root is used to treat rheumatism and syphilis in Russia. The juice of berries is given in affection of the respiratory passage. The plant yields two alkaloids, ephedrine and pseudoephedrine. Ephedrine has the property of dilating the pupil of the eye. Liquid extract is used in asthma and tincture is used as a cardiac and circulatory stimulant. In China the stem is considered diaphoretic and antipyretic and the root is used as a mild astringent. The root is considered alterative, stomachic; and tonic.

Claviceps purpurea. This is a fungus (commonly known as Ergot) which grows as a parasite on some cereals. It contains a number of toxic alkaloids including ergotamine, ergotaxin, ergometrine and lysergice acid. It stimulates involuntary muscles in the body and interferes with the production and distribution of adrenalin. Ergometrine acts mainly on the muscles of the uterus by contracting and thus reducing the blood loss after birth. Ergotamine constricts small blood vessels in the head and counteracts migraine.

Some Important Medicinal Plants in Kenya

Kenya is rich in herbal medicine and a very large number of species are used as traditional medicines (Kokwaro, 1976; 1988). Virtually every plant has some or other use. Some families of flowering plants are noted for their therapeutic value and various drugs of great medicinal importance have been extracted. However, in a chapter like this, it is not possible to discuss all such herbs and, therefore, a few important ones have been chosen arbitrarily belonging to three important families of flowering plants namely, *Solanaceae, Apocyanaceae* and *Leguminoceae*.

Many medicinal herbs are highly poisonous and, if used in large dosages may prove fatal to livestock as well as humans. Some plants may have only some specific parts with poisonous properties such as fruits or seeds (as in some apocyanaceous or euphorbiaceous seeds). Reports of contact poisoning in adults and in children who happened to eat it unknowingly, appear frequently. For example, castor oil plant (*Ricinus communis*), belonging to the family of euphorbiaceae and which is quite common in Kenya growing along roadsides or in cultivated fields, is used as an effective cure for constipation. The oil is safe but the seeds are extremely poisonous — a dosage of only one or two seeds may cause death. When the oil is extracted the poisonous substances called recin (belonging to the poisonous protein compound toxalbumin) is left behind.

The family Solanaceae

The family solanaceae is especially known for plants of medicinal value such as the deadly nightshade, the thorn apple, the henbane and *solanum* sp.

Two species of thorn apple (*Datura*) have been reported to be used as herbal medicine in Kenya, namely D. *metel* and D. *stramonium*. The extract of *Datura* is often used as an intoxicant having a feeling of alcohol which, if taken in large quantities, may cause severe headache, drowsiness or even unconsciousness. The decoction is inhaled in asthma but it enhances the bronchial condition. The alkaloid has similar symptoms as belladone.

Many species of the genus *Solanum* such as potato and egg plant are medicinally important besides their economic importance as crop plants. More than ten species of this genus are used in Kenya by traditional healers to cure various ailments (Kokwaro, 1976). The root decoction of *S. incanum* is used for abdominal pain, fever and indigestion. The species *S. dasyphyllum* is used for curing hookworm; the boiled root is taken internally and the crushed leaves taken against stomach troubles. The species *S. aculeastrum* is used to treat bronchitis and gonorrhoea while the leaves of *S. goetzel* are used externally as poultice on swellings and abscesses. *S. nigrium* is well known for its medicinal use in Asia and Africa and the leaves, fruits and seeds are all medicinally important. Pounded leaves, soaked and fermented, and fruits are used as a cure for boils, stomachache, ulcers and swollen glands.

Withania somnifera is another species of this family reputed for its medicinal use. The roots, pounded or boiled, are used as a cure for gastric ulcers, skin rashes, gonorrhoea and different types of pains. Fine ground and dried powder of roots is also taken with honey against cold.

The boiled roots of *Lycium europaeum* are also taken as a medicine for colds and coughs.

The family Apocyanaceae

Another family of flowering plants which is noted for its medicinal properties is *Apocyanaceae* although most of the plants of this family are highly poisonous. Such include *Acocanthera longifolia*, *Acocanthera schimperi, Catharanthus roseus, Thevetia peruviana, Narium oleander, Strophanthus kombe, Desvaux-Holarrhena pubescens* and *Rauwolfia serpentina.*

Acocanthera longifolia and *A. schimperi* are known to be useful against syphillis and possess cardiac glycoside. These species are however highly poisonous to livestock and man and have been reported to be used as arrow poison during tribal conflicts since stone age and therefore ought to be taken with great caution.

Rauwolfia serpentina is a universally accepted drug and contains many alkaloid. It is highly effective in controlling high blood pressure. In Kenya three species of *Rauwolfia*, namely *R. caffra*, *R. mombasiana* and *R. vomitoria*, have been reported to be used in traditional medicine. The root and bark decoction is used against rheumatic pain and fever.

Holarrhena febrifuga leaves, pounded with water, are used against stomachache. The roots are febrifuge and are used to bathe children to reduce fever.

Strophanthus kombe of coastal Kenya, is a climber with yellowish-white flowers with red splashes and a long tail. The fruits are pods which grow in pairs. It has a cardiac glycoside, strophanthin, which is not as poisonous as oleandrin and ouabain. It has similar effects as digitalin from *Digitalis purpurea* and is used in mild doses to help stabilize a weak heart. It is also highly poisonous and, if taken in large quantities, may prove to be fatal because the heart fails to keep pumping.

Strophanthus eminii is also used as a febrifuge to bathe children having high fever. The root is emetic; its decoction is given internally to exterminate worms. Seeds are highly poisonous and are used as arrow poison.

Nerium oleander and *Thevetia peruviana* are both highly poisonous plants with cardiac glycosides, oleandrin and thevatin respectively. All contacts with any part of fruit, bark, root or milky juice is recommended to be avoided.

Adenium obesum and *A. somalense* of this family are also highly poisonous and are used as arrow and fish poison by certain ethnic groups in East Africa. They contain the substances Saponina and sapotoxin which, though not so poisonous for the warm blooded animals, may sometimes prove to be quite dangerous in other cases.

The root decoction of *Carissa edulis* of this family is used to relieve pain and indigestion and to cure malaria.

The family Leguminosae

The family leguminosae has a large number of species of medicinal importance. Specially worth mentioning is the genus *Cassia* with many species such as *C. abbreviata*, *C. didymobotrya*, *C. floribuda*, *C. mimosoides*, *C. occidentalis*, *C. senna* and *C. singueana*. The *Cassia* leaves, dried and made into powder, are used as purgative in constipation and as antihelminthic to remove worms. Besides stomach ailment they are also at times used for other ailments including fever, malaria, gonorrhoea and syphilis.

Extracts of *Cassia senna* have been in use as laxative and purgative for hundreds of years. It is not very poisonous, but when taken in large doses, it may cause diarrhoea and excessive dehydration which may lead to death in some cases. The laxative property is due to a compound called anthraquinone.

Tamarindus indica, a tree found in the dry coastal region of Kenya, is used in treating diarrhoea and dysentery. A root decoction is drunk against cough and fever. The fruit is carminative, laxative, refrigeranate and in fabrile diseases. The fruit contains traces of oxalic acid.

Some species of *Acacia*, especially their barks, are used for treating cough and sore throat, for example, *A. gerrardii*. The infusion of the root of *A. brevispica* is used to remove intestinal worms.

The red water tree (*Erythrophlem suaveolens*) is known to be an ordeal poison and has been used as arrow poison and rat poison besides having medicinal properties. It has cardiac glycosides such as erythrophlamine and erythrophleine, which cause vomiting, diarrhoea, thirst and headache. The leaves were used in tribal ordeal to judge the innocence of a culprit as it was believed that a person was innocent if he could stand the medicine without showing any of those symptoms. Root decoction is used as antihelminthic and ametic to exterminate tape worms. The other species, *E. africanum*, is used as a purgative.

The extract of *Dichrostachys cinerea* leaves is used to treat stomachaches and conjunctivitis. The root, bark and leaves are all medically important with the root decoction being used in scorpion bites and considered an aphrodisiac.

Abrus precatorius and *A. schimperi* are used both as an aphrodisiac and against stomachache and the leaves are used in scorpion bites. The seeds are toxic however. Paste of seeds is applied externally as a rubifacient in sciatica, stiff shoulders, paralysis and other nervous disorders. The root is considered demulcent, emetic and elexiteric.

Piliostigma thonningii, known as *mchikichiki* in Kiswahili, is commonly used as a medicinal herb in Kenya. Its leaves, roots, bark and juice are all medicinally important. The green leaves and the juice are taken to treat stomachache. The root infusion is taken as a remedy against colds and venereal diseases and to stop bleeding and miscarriage in women.

Some species of this leguminosae family are also used by medicinemen in witchcraft and are considered superstitious. These include *Entada abyssinica, Leucaena leucocephala* and *Cajanus cajan* which are supposed to bring good omen or counteract witchcraft.

Mode of Traditional Herbal Therapy

Most of the medicinal herbs are poisonous if taken in large quantities. Therefore, the dosage should be prepared with great care and accuracy. Unless a chemical analysis is done, it may not be possible to estimate the exact quantity of the extract that can be used as the correct dose; any additional amount may cause deleterious symptoms or even death. However, traditional healers, with their long practical experience, are well versed in their estimate of dosage.

The active medicinal principles, especially the glycosides, alkoloids, asteroids, oils and fats are said to be the agents which have curative properties. Under different climatic and ecological conditions, the active principles in plants may vary at different stages of their development. Not only do they vary at different times of the season, but also in different parts of the same plant. It has been reported that the essential oil in mints (*Mentha* sp.) varies at different levels of the plant from the gound (i.e., at the top, middle and lower part of the same plant).

Herbal medicines are prepared and administered in different ways. Usually it may be given in the form of infusion, crude liquid extract or hot decoction of the whole herb or its parts, such as flowers, seeds, leaves, root, bark or gum. The whole plant or its part may be soaked in water overnight or pounded and boiled. The crude extract or decoction thus obtained may be given internally or applied externally as poultice to the affected part such as skin eruption, lesions or wounds. A summary of different methods used is given below:

Leaves– Infusion of leaves is used as bath. Leaves are passed through steam and vapour inhaled to cure fever.

Leaves are heated over fire and applied as poultice over the wound, rashes or enlarged glands.

Leaves are powdered with water or crushed and applied as poultice.

Leaves are chewed and juice swallowed.

Leaves are boiled and the decoction drunk to cure various ailments.

Leaves are smoked.

Leaves are employed as an inhalent for fever.

The vapour from crushed leaves is inhaled for treatment of fever.

Root– Roots are pounded and the juice is rubbed as an antidote to general poisoning.

Roots are boiled and decoction taken.

Roots are pounded and mixed with castor oil and taken.

Roots are cooked with meat or vegetable and the soup is drunk.

Roots are seeped in cold water and the liquid is drunk.

Roots are ground to powder and applied on wounds and rashes.

Stem –Young branches are roasted and chewed.

Seed – Seeds are ground and mixed with vegetable fat and the paste applied on sores.

Fruit – Fruits are crushed and soaked in hot water overnight and drunk.

Bulb –Paste prepared from bulb is used to dress wounds or earache.

Latex –Milky latex or sap of some herbs is used for the treatment of hookworm.

Bark –The bark of both stem and roots are usually used in the same way as the leaves, as mentioned above.

Conclusion

In some parts of the world, traditional medicine has been recognized and patronized by the government and a systematic screening of medicinal plants has begun in specialized institutions. However, in many other countries, there still exists some scepticism about the merits of the traditional medical system.

The authenticity of the claims about the medicinal value of some herbs has been scientifically tested and many are exploited commercially. However, a large number of these herbs that are traditionally used are yet to be verified using modern pharmacological and pharmaceutical techniques. The problems involved in their exploitation — from their raw state to the pilot plant scale and to industry stage, is not an easy one especially if the standardization of the drug is considered. Some suggestions on the exploitation of such useful herbs has been published elsewhere (Baquar, 1991). Emphasis has been made on a thorough survey as the first logical step followed by a series of steps to be taken towards standardization of the drug.

Each medicinal herb has to be studied botanically, pharcognostically, chemically and clinically. The life history of each species will also have to be ascertained from the germination to the harvest stage under different ecological conditions to know the range of various qualitative and quantitative diversity at different stages of plant growth. The active principles, which are confined to the cortical cells, barks, roots, stem, leaves, flowers, fruits or seeds, will have to be correctly traced by anatomical, micro-chemical or chemical tests. The periodicity of the individual species will also have to be worked out in order to find out when the active principles reach their optimum in the plant and are most efficacious.

Though the "botanical affluence" of the tropical plant species has been recognized by many institutions in Africa, the number of research publications by African scientists on African plant species is relatively low (Abegaz, 1991).

The tropical ecosystems, however, are being destroyed at an alarmingly high rate; it is estimated that by the year 2000, approximately 20-25 per cent of the plant species is likely to be destroyed (Raghavan, 1991). There is, therefore, need to develop a mechanism to protect these species by evolving internationally recognized policies for the management of plant resources, especially the species of medicinal value.

The future of drugs depends, to a great extent, on the study of natural sources of remedies. The vast unexplored herbal medicines may ultimately provide remedies to scores of our ailments.

REFERENCES

Abegaz, B. 1991. *Science Policies and Natural Product Research in Africa. 4th NAPRECA Symposium on Natural Products*. pp.1-4 (Dec. 16-21), Addis Ababa, Ethiopia.

Baquar, S. R. 1989. *Medicinal Poisonous Plants of Pakistan*. Karachi: Printas Ltd.

__________. 1991. Indigenous Medicinal Herbs and their Exploitation" *Sinet Newsletter* (24(3):4-8.

Baquar, S. R. and M. Tasnif. 1967. *Medicinal Plants of Southern West Pakistan.* PCSIR Monograph No. 3, Karachi:

Koinange, W. 1982. *Health Strategy for Kenya.* Nairobi: Ministry of Health.

Kokwaro, J. O. 1976. *Medicinal Plants of East Africa:* Nairobi: East African Literature Bureau.

Kokwaro, J. O. 1988. "Traditional Methods of Treating Skin Diseases in Kenya Through the Use of Plants." *Monogr. Syst. Bot. Missouri Bo. Gard.* 25:363-372.

Lehane, B. 1977. *The Power of Plants.* Mainenhead, Eng.: McGraw Hill.

Raghavan, C. 1991. *The West Australian.* 24th March, 1991.

Chapter 13

MANAGEMENT OF MEDICINAL PLANT RESOURCES IN NYANZA

Opportunities for Crop Renewal and Promising Conservation Strategies

E. A. Ochieng' Obado and J. A. Odera

Introduction

Like pastoralists in different parts of Africa, the people of Nyanza Province possess a very intimate knowledge of the characteristics and values of different plants. They can recognise those plants that are toxic to human beings and animals; those

- which stimulate milk and meat production in livestock;
- with salty characteristics;
- which indicate the agricultural potential of different soils, habitats or ecosystems;
- which produce various types of wood products; and,
- with medicinal potential for man and livestock (Spencer, 1965).

But the extent and depth of this knowledge base varies among different communities.

It is also evident that a lot is known about food, medicinal herbs and plants with toxic properties while there is virtually no information on protocols for their sustainable management, including when or how to harvest, methods of regeneration or cultivation of these plants. In the past, with large areas of bushland, forest fallow and open community land lying within easy reach of the villages, this omission was of little significance. Consequently, the pioneer botanists and naturalists have been preoccupied with describing the major flora, and in a few cases, have recognized medicinal potentials of different plants for managing given ailments (Watt and Breyer - Brandwijk, 1962; Verdcourt and Trump, 1969; Kokwaro, 1976). In a few cases supportive chemical studies have provided information on chemical compounds of pharmacological or therapeutic value with some focus on opportunities of obtaining clues on potential bases for modern industrial drugs (Morton, 1977; Swain, 1972). Currently, the field has become very attractive with a growing body of literature documenting plant species of medicinal value used in different parts of the country.

It is to be noted, however, that what once appeared as inexhaustible sources of herbal medicine and other products has since greatly diminished as a result of population pressure and increasing demand for land for agriculture and settlement. This has been exacerbated by the consequences of land adjudication and consolidation under individual ownership, resulting in intensive use of farmlands with virtually no fallow period. Regretfully, this is happening at a time when more and more people are turning to traditional medicine, partly as a result of the escalating cost of allopathic medicine and partly as a consequence of renewed interest in traditional values. It is estimated that between 75 and 90 per cent of the population in Africa rely in one way or other on herbal medicine (Falconer, 1990; Ayensu, 1983). A recent survey by the Kenya Forestry Research Institute (KEFRI) shows that over 90 per cent of Kenyans use medicinal plants. However, this could be an underestimation if the number of those who visit traditional healers secretly (due to personal reasons) is taken into account.

In response to this growing demand for and interest in traditional medicine, a number of African governments have recognized the importance of ethnomedical practice and encouraged it together with modern medical care (Falconer, 1990). However, the benefits of traditional medicine can only be maintained and developed if the supply of the medicinal plants can be assured and sustained. Understandably, the way the target plants are harvested, regenerated and conserved will determine the future of traditional medicine.

Historically, development and deforestation have gone hand in hand. It is estimated that every year 36,000 hectares (ha) of indigenous forests are lost in Kenya alone (Redfern, 1992) due to the rising demand for wood products and the expansion of agriculture and settlements. Moreover, the existing policy addressing conservation through the development of forests, wildlife and game reserves cannot cater for the diversity of medicinal plant species that are scattered in different habitats. This is because forest and wildlife reservations tend to be ecologically restricted.

But under existing land use practices, the gazetted forests and game parks as well as the related biosphere reserves, covering only 11 per cent of the country, are the only visible secure depositories of indigenous biotic wealth. In many districts, especially in Nyanza Province, where there are no such reserves, the residual vegetation found in different ecosystems in trust-land areas or private fields are the only remaining depositories of valuable plant genetic resources that the province can count on.

Also, with continued loss of natural vegetation and forests around the villages, herbalists, vendors and those others who rely on traditional medicine are forced to travel long distances to obtain medicinal plant material and hence the resultant hikes in prices. The need for assuring a stable and sustainable resource base of medicinal plants is therefore an urgent and indeed imperative task.

This chapter reports the results of a study undertaken over a period of one year in Nyanza Province. Among other tasks, the study focused on documenting and appraising:

(i) the major medicinal plants used for common ailments;
(ii) harvesting practices and methods used by main stakeholders with a view to assessing their sustainability;
(iii) renewal methods frequently used; and,
(iv) opportunities for conserving endangered plant germplasm.

The visits and interviews covered a total of 128 homes and 45 traditional healers in the six districts of Nyanza Province (Table 13.1). In addition, discussions were held with herbalists and vendors who sell medicinal plant material at Kibuye market in Kisumu, and markets in Homa Bay, Siaya and Kisii towns. Visual assessment of different aspects of land use was made through windscreen surveys and during visits to homes, research stations and on-farm plots. The results reported here are based on information accumulated during these interviews and drawn from anecdotal and oral qualitative evidence collected.

The Study Area

The area under discussion is Nyanza Province. It is not endowed with much forest cover. Pockets of natural forest and vegetation are found in Kisii and South Nyanza Districts. Islands of game reserves are found in South Nyanza; Ruma

Table 13.1: Families and traditional healers visited in Nyanza Province

Area/District	Families (No.)	Traditional healers (No.)
Kisii and Nyamira	12	2
Homa Bay and Migori	30	10
Kuria	6	0
Kisumu	45	15
Siaya	35	18
Total	128	45

National Park, the largest of these is about 12,000 ha. Afforestation in Kisii was started under the African Land Development (ALDEV) programme in 1953 when a forester was posted to the district to provide advisory services. In the rest of the province, forest extension work was started in 1971 for Kisumu District, 1972 for South Nyanza (now divided into Migori, Homa Bay and Kuria Districts) and 1975 for Siaya District under the rural afforestation extention scheme. But the impact of forest extension remained marginal until 1986 when foresters were deployed to all administrative divisions of the province; while technicians were deployed to the locations to develop nurseries and advise farmers on tree growing. It is evident that in the whole of Nyanza Province, the forest department stáff have hitherto concentrated on raising exotic species, such as cypress, eucalyptus and pines. Only a few indigenous tree species are raised. No deliberate attempt has been made to incorporate any of the useful medicinal plants in the afforestation programme. Noticeably, little attempt has been made to advise farmers on methods of conserving medicinal herbs and plants of cultural importance.

The population density in the study area varies from an average of 250 persons per square kilometer in the dry areas to 430 persons per square kilometre in the wetter zones. Similarly, rainfall varies from an annual average of 700 mm in the dry parts to about 1800 mm in the wetter areas. The economy in Kisii and Nyamira Districts is mainly focused on intensive agricultural crop production while in the other districts, the residents practise mixed farming with an emphasis on indigenous cattle rearing.

Results

Traditional medicine

This component of the study examined access to medicinal plants by the communities and the sustainability of the sources. In the course of the interviews, it became evident that what was defined as "within easy reach" or available in the "distant horizon" varied and depended on the three major informal categories of resource users. For purposes of this discussion, these categories of users have been grouped into the following three according to economies of scale and levels of specialisation:

(a) the immediate family source:
(b) the family's traditional physician; and,
(c) the professional healers (magicians, herbalists and so on).

Out of the 128 families interviewed, all appeared to have some working information on herbal medicine for common ailments and diseases. For instance, among the Luo, a common herb *Ageratum conyzoides (oluoro chieng')* is widely used in treating fresh wounds to stop bleeding and for treating swollen bruises. *Leonotis* sp. *(nyanyodhi)* is used for treating abdominal pain, while *Aloe sp.* is used for managing poultry diseases. The bark of common medicinal plant species such as *Fagara macrophylla (sogo-maitha), Zanthoxylum usambarense (roko),* and *Toddalia asiatica (nyalwetkwach)* are kept by members of the family for emergency home use. Many common ailments including coughs, measles, colds, constipation/indigestion, worms, diarrhoea, abdominal pains, headache, sprains and cattle diseases are tackled on an emergency basis at family level.

Most families reported that they visited hospitals, veterinarians and traditional healers only when the family's physician failed. Many cases where clinical medicine failed were referred to the family physician or professional healers. Teachers and religious leaders were generally reluctant to admit ever using traditional treatments, but they often revealed knowledge of the uses of plants and the diseases treated. This observation conflicts with their denial.

In general, women were found to be more conversant with herbal medicine than their male counterparts. It seems that the division of labour, where women are close to the children and manage the household, favours this development. Moreover, the majority of the women interviewed acknowledged that they had learnt healing skills from their mothers, grandmothers and female friends. Surprisingly, even the men who were knowledgeable on medicinal plants appear to have acquired more information from their mothers than from their fathers.

The Luo family traditional physician (*ajuoga*) is largely a herbalist who rarely mixes plant material with other accompaniments. But animal products such as fats and droppings may be added where appropriate. He is often a specialist in a narrow spectrum of disease conditions. Such knowledge often runs in families although the information can be passed outside the family network on payment of a handsome fee. Cases where specialist traditional physicians have become generalist healers are not rare. Professional traditional healers acquire their skills through inheritance, apprenticeship or internship. The majority are possessed with "spirits" of their ancestors or mentors who of necessity were healers during their time. Practitioners in this category publicly acknowledge the powers of their trainers and claim to be guided by spirits of departed relatives who visit them, during a trance or through visions, to direct them on prescriptions of specific plants for treating different conditions, particularly new and challenging cases.

Sources of medicinal plant material

Medicinal plant material used at the family level is largely drawn from the homestead, the home garden and from fallows, thickets and woodlands within a locus of three kilometre radius from the village. *Euphorbia tirucalli* live fences provide rich niches and habitats for many important herbs, arthropods, amphibians, small reptiles, birds and small mammals. Despite private ownership rights associated with land adjudication and registration, medicinal plants are still collected from neighbour's fields without any restrictions or hindrance. But cultivated plants can only be harvested with permission of the owner.

Quite often, members of the family do not travel long distances to obtain their herbs; but raw materials of key medicinal plants are often passed on by friends or relatives living in areas close to habitats of such plants. Some materials are purchased from reputed markets, but in this instance the knowledgeable member of the family purchases a specific plant material that he/she uses for the given complaint. But there are increasing cases where individuals seek advice from vendors in the open market on medicinal plants for given complaints and then buy the recommended materials. The homestead hedge is a rich source of medicinal plants.

During the survey, an attempt was made to assess the occurrence, and distribution of key plants along alleys in agroforestry trails, fallows, bushlands, woodlots and the live homestead hedge. This study was undertaken because of the growing popularity of alley farming in extension circles, the rapidly shrinking areas of open land and the increasing use of exotic species for live fences. Observations from ground survey had revealed that many families in the province surrounded their homesteads with *E. tirucalli* hedges. The hedge is often allowed to grow to its maximum height of about 8 meters and generally dies due to senescence after 15 to 18 years. However, a few families have introduced *Cupressus lusitanica* and *Dovyalis caffra* live hedges.

Results of numerical counts of occurrence of the major species, in association with these habitats in different agroclimatic zones, show that the larger species diversity is associated with *E. tirucalli* hedge than in the other habitats examined. Over 22 species of medicinal plants were found growing in association with an *E. tirucalli* hedge in one homestead in Asembo location in Siaya District.

Distribution and marketing of medicinal plants

A number of medicinal plants are available in market centres, especially in

Kisumu. These include *Fagara macrophylla (sogo maitha), Warbugia ugandensis (abaki), Mitragyna stipulosa (obul)* and *Acanthus* sp. (*seje*). The majority of users are unable to recognize these plants in the wild although they expressed keenness to plant them.

Professional or semi-professional herbalists and traditional healers in general maintain a shroud of secrecy on the source of plant materials that they prescribe. It was apparent that preference is accorded to plants from the sub-humid areas *vis-a-vis* plants from the high potential areas of wet lands, except in a few specific cases where trees from the wet habitats may be preferred. Some herbalists claimed that the source of the plant material that they use in each case is revealed by the spirits during the examination of the patient. A herbalist who specialises in treating cases of mental disease observed that he often travels to sites in Uganda and the Coast Province, about 600 kilometres from his base in Kisumu, to procure specific plant material. It was not clear whether during such visits, they obtain the medicinal plant material from a reputable site on their own or obtain it from a knowledgeable local herbalist. Many herbalists maintained that success in curing certain diseases depended on their ability to obtain potent materials from specific sources and their skills in the preparation of decoctions, a process that involves stewing different plant materials together in given proportions. According to a Kamba medicineman who sells medicinal plant material at Kibuye market in Kisumu, *Sclerocarya birrea* (*ong'ono adhiang'*) from Nyanza is more potent in treating cases of snake bites than material grown

13.2: Some Common medicinal plant species marketed in Kisumu town but harvested from outside the Province

Species	Source area
Alstonia boonei	Uganda, Busia
Azadirachta indica	Coast
Artemisia afra	Nakuru District
Ekebergia rueppelliana	Nairobi and Rift valley Province
Fagara macrophylla	Kericho and Kakamega
Jateorhiza palmata	Coast
Khaya senegalensis	Uganda
Ocotea usambarensis	Nairobi and Central Province
Pappea guinensis	Kakamega
Pappea capensis	Kakamega
Rauwolfia caffra	Kericho
Warburgia ugandensis	Nairobi

in Machakos District. This view was shared by other vendors of medicinal plants at Kibuye. Another example that was volunteered by the vendors was *Pappea guinensis* where root samples from Kakamega appeared to be more bitter to taste than those from Busia and were regarded as more effective. But certain species such as *Fagara macrophylla, Chlorophora exelsa*, and *Warbugia ugandensis* are said to be effective regardless of their origin. Table 13.2 summarises some common plant species that are sold at Kibuye market.

FAO (1986) reports variations in reserpine content in *Rauwolfia vomitoria* growing in Congo, which contains up to 10 times more reserpine than that grown in neighbouring Uganda.

Harvesting Practices and Erosion of Plant Genetic Resources

Although leaves and branches of plants are often used in the preparation of different decoctions, the popular practice gives preference for roots and mature bark of woody plants while whole plants are used for less woody plants. The extraction of the whole tree to harvest the roots is a popular practice in harvesting medicinal plants (Table 13.3). But in a few cases, only a small fraction of the roots was removed leaving the plant with a good chance for survival. People harvesting the roots of *Carissa edulis (achuoga)* and *Teclea nobilis (odar)* were obliged by custom to return the soil to cover the remaining roots. The Luo believe that if the hole is left open, one's enemy could later remove the remaining roots and use these to bewitch the user.

Table 13.3: Some important species harvested by uprooting the whole plant

Species	Parts used
Achyranthus aspera	roots, stems and leaves
Artemisia afra	roots
Calotropis procera	roots
Carissa edulis	roots
Cassia didymobotrya	roots, stem bark, leaves
Cassia occidentalis	roots, leaves
Capparis erythrocarpos	roots
Entada abyssinica	roots, bark and leaves
Maerua edulis	tuber
Ocimum basilicum	roots, stems and leaves
Solanum incanum	roots, leaves and fruits
Tecona stans	roots, bark and leaves

Although there are strong taboos against cutting certain sacred trees, there does not appear to be any traditional belief or practice that forestalls or mitigates destructive exploitation or over-use of medicinal plants among the Luo. The popular method of harvesting medicinal plants by extracting whole plants is wasteful, destructive and non-sustainable. Consequently, a number of popular medicinal plants such as *Capparis erythrocarpos (ong'ono)* and *Maerua edulis (amoyo)*, a versatile medicinal plant with edible tubers, are currently severely endangered. The four species used for managing cattle diseases, *Staganotaenia araliacea (niang liach)* and *Erythrina abyssinica (murembe), Ormocarpum trichocarpum (det)*, and *Boscia salicifolia (okado-maracher),* have become extremely rare as well due to heavy harvesting pressures involving extraction of whole trees. Fortunately, some of the species listed on table 13.3 such as *Occium basilium (mueny), Solanum incanum (ochok)* and *Achyranthus aspera (ayucha)* regenerate profusely either through seed or by coppicing.

Both men and women trade in medicinal plant material. Table, 13.4 shows that out of 40 vendors interviewed on one market day at Kibuye, the majority had come from Kisumu; but one had come from Nandi, two from Machakos and four from Busia.

Table 13.4: Source origin of medicinal plants by district

Districts of origin	Number of vendors marketing the medicinal plants
Nandi	1
Machakos	2
Kakamega	5
Busia	4
Siaya	7
South Nyanza	5
Kisumu	16
Total	40

These results differ slightly from those reported by Sindiga (1992) from surveys done in Narok District whereby he observes that the majority of people using medicinal plants in Narok District rely on plants harvested within the district with only a minority collecting material from outside. It is probable that this difference arises from the higher concentrations of indigenous forests in the district compared to any of the districts in Nyanza.

Another destructive method of harvesting observed during the survey involves the peeling of the bark of growing trees. Table 13.5 lists some species grown in Kenyan forests for timber and other purposes that have been recorded either partially or totally ring-barked for harvesting the bark for medicinal use (C.f. Kokwaro, 1976).

Table 13.5: Valuable forest timber species found in Kenyan forests partially or fully ring-barked for herbal medicine

Species	Common names	Uses
*Afzelia quanzensis**	*mbambakofi*— Swahili	Used for cattle diseases, snake bite and chest pains.
Bischoffia javanica	bishopwood	Stomach problems, diarrhoea
Chlorophora excelsa	*mvule* - Swahili olua - Luo	Rheumatic fever, cough, heart problem.
*Cordia africana**	*muririga* - Swahili; *mukoma* - Luhya	Livestock diseases and for tying broken bones
*Dalbergia melanoxylon**	African ebony - *mpingo* - Swahili	Treating worms and abdominal pains
Ekebergia rueppeliana	*mununga* - Kikuyu *tido* - Luo	Chest pains, cattle diseases
Fagara macrophylla	*sogowait* - Kipsigis; *sogomaitha* - Luo	Constipation, snake bite rheumatic fever.
Hagenia abyssinica	*mumondo* - Kikuyu	Diarrhoea and stomach ache
Khaya senegalensis	mahogany	Malaria fever, venereal diseases and livestock diseases.
Olea welwitschii	*Loliondo* - Luganda; *mutukufu* - Luhya	Venereal diseases and stomach ache
Ocotea usambarensis	camphor	Cancer, boils, back ache, cough, livestock diseases
Podocarpus milanjianus	podo	Stomach ache and Cattle diseases
Podocarpus gracilior	podo	Stomach ache and cattle diseases
Prunus africanum	*mueri* –Kikuyu *munyama*- Luhya	Stomach ache and cattle diseases
Trichilia emetica	*mururi* - Kikuyu *munyama* - Luhya	Diarrhoea and chest pains
Warburgia ugandensis	*muthiga* - Kikuyu *abaki* - Luo	Chest pains, muscle pains, weak joints.

* Status: Endangered

In the farmlands, harvesting of the bark is widespread on bushes and fallows, a practise largely perpetrated by the owners of the holdings. This was surprising because where a user is harvesting medicinal plant raw materials from trees in his own field, given the security of tenure, it is logical to expect him to harvest conservatively, allowing the tree a good chance to recover and provide more raw materials in future. In contrast, the family physician and the professional healers observe particular care in harvesting raw materials from their plant resources. This perhaps reflects a higher level of professional ethics.

Popular species affected by destructive harvesting in the farmlands are presented on Table 13.6. Trees which are heavily or totally ring-barked die within one to two seasons. It is not clear whether ring-barking is done in ignorance of its effect on the life of the tree or driven by selfish motives in defiance of the needs for sustainability. Some herbalists contend that mature bark on the main stem has more potent alkaloids.

Kokwaro (1988) has suggested that herbalists harvesting medicinal plants in Kakamega forest should be asked to remove small pieces of bark from several trees instead of removing large quantities of bark from a few favourites. He estimates that there are enough trees of favoured species to allow for the removal of small pieces of bark.

However, the removal of the bark exposes the tree to the risk of attack by pests and diseases thereby reducing the commercial value of the species. Other methods of harvesting observed include cutting the whole stem and harvesting leaves, flowers and fruits. Harvesting leaves and fruits was found to be the safest and ecologically least destructive method used in Nyanza.

Table 13.6: Some tree species in Nyanza found in farms partially or fully ring-barked for herbal medicines

Botanical Name	Luo Name
Albizia coriara	*ober*
Azadirachta indica	*nim (nyamin dwelle)*
Bridelia micrantha	*athuno*
Cassia siamea	*oyieko*
Chlorophora excelsa	*mvule, olua*
Commiphora africana	*arupiny*
Gardenia lutea	*rayudhi*
Lannea stuhlmanni	*kwoyo*
Mitragyana stipulosa	*obul*
Sclerocarya birrea	*ongono adhiang'*
Warburgia ugandensis	*abaki*

It has also been proposed that harvesting of medicinal woody plants should be restricted to the bark of branches to be drawn by pollarding. However, this option is unlikely to be enforced unless it is established that the variations in the composition and concentration of chemical compounds between branches and the main stem are not significant. Because harvesting by pollarding of branches provides scope for sustainable management, appropriate research should be undertaken to address this concern.

Propagation and Conservation of Medicinal Plants

Results of windscreen surveys carried out in all districts in Nyanza Province clearly showed that many exotic tree species, such as *Cassia siamea, Eucalyptus, Grevellia robusta* and mangoes have become important components of the landscape. Traditional healers have also played a leading role in planting species such as *Alstonia boonei, Cassia siamea, Delonix ragia, Eucalyptus citrodora, Melia azedarach, Tecoma stans, Thevestia peruviana* and *Tilhonia diversifolia.* However, traditional healers generally advised the community, particularly their clients, against planting certain species such as *Jatropha curcas (jok), Blighia unijugata (bilo), Erythrina abyssinica (murembe), Plumbago zeylanica (rachier), Caesalpinia volkensii (ajua)* and several species of *Euphorbia* and *Aloe* in their homesteads, least they are struck by bad luck. However, it is to be noted that professional healers often conserve these in hidden corners within their holdings. Traditionally, certain sacred trees, such as *Chlorophora excelsa (mvule)* and *E. abyssinica* are not supposed to be planted. They generally regenerate on their own. It is taboo to cut such trees. Mvule is only cut on full awareness of members of the clan, following an appropriate sacrificial offering to the ancestors.

Generally, many traditional healers travel long distances to obtain medicinal plant parts where tree species do not occur nearby, or where they have good reason to recognise varietal differences. Some traditional healers maintain medicinal plant groves, bushlands and fallows which they use as a source of medicinal plants. These sites are generally revered or dreaded by the local people. No cutting or grazing takes place in such places for fear of meeting a definite retribution or sudden death. One traditional healer in Siaya District grows many introduced species of herbs and shrubs. He confided that he had learnt of the medicinal value of some exotic plants which he cultivates in his home garden from an Asian friend.

Another traditional healer in Nyakach Location in Kisumu District was also found growing different herbs and shrubs in a small home-garden that was well protected by a live fence. These two examples are a step in the right direction in conserving the valuable plant genetic resources. This may well form a nucleus for developing user-driven conservation strategies in the future.

Discussion and Conclusion

Observations made during this study reveal that thickets, bushland, fallows, forests and savanna woodlands that once provided a kingdom for a wide range of medicinal plants are shrinking rapidly due to increasing population pressure and associated developmental activities. This has led to the loss of biodiversity including important medicinal plants. Many popular medicinal plant species, such as *Capparis erythrocarpus (ong'ono), Steganotania araliacea (niang liech),* and *Maerea edulis (amoyo)*, are threatened as a result of destructive methods of harvesting, over-exploitation and absence of a renewable (regeneration) programme. Indeed, no seedlings of medicinal plants were found in any of the nurseries in the province. This is surprising because the current tree planting agenda is largely preoccupied with raising plants for fuelwood and agro-forestry species.

This study also shows that there is an urgent need to incorporate programmes on *ex-situ* and *in-situ* conservation of medicinal plants in the agenda on conservation and sustainable management of plant genetic resources in the province. This calls for integrating the efforts of traditional healers and members of local communities in drawing land use plans on the management of bushlands, savannas, woodlands and forests in their immediate environs. All conservation efforts should focus on managing whole ecosystems or forest types as this would sustain the full richness of plant and animal life. In contrast, attempts to realise specific programmes for individual plants would be prohibitive and inadequate in scope to cater for biodiversity.

Destructive harvesting methods practised by individual families, traditional physicians, professional healers and vendors imputes lack of concern for sustainability. This is probably a consequence of past abundance of indigenous plant germplasm and community land ownership.

Certain harvesting techniques are depleting herbal resources. This is the case with harvesting of the whole tree which is endangering many plant species such as *Steganotania araliacea* and *Erythrina abyssinica*. Harvesting of roots is also a very destructive method because it leads to instant death of the plant. Ring-barking is also a method of harvesting which should be discouraged through sensitising the stake holders of its consequences on resource sustainability. The possibility of using the bark from branches instead of the main stem should be explored.

It is recommended that scientists and stakeholders should:

develop non-destructive and conservative cropping regimes, such as harvesting of renewable components of plants including pollarding of branches, plucking of leaves, removal of small proportions of lateral roots and on each occasion replacing the soil to protect the remaining root systems.

encourage responsible government departments to establish a licensing system that allows for controlled harvesting of medicinal plants to be monitored through inspection and certification.

In terms of research and development, there is an urgent need to mount a programme on surveys on traditional medicines and plant species used for different medical conditions. Such surveys would establish baseline data, assess what is being lost and devise meaningful strategies for conservation and opportunities for sustainable use of target plant resources. Finally, a monitoring system is required for assessing changes in biodiversity. Another area is to examine possible variations in the concentrations of the active ingredients in the foliage, floral parts, branches, barks of younger and older stem and the roots; between different site conditions and seasons of the year. The potentials of indigenous technologies, such as the live *E. tirucalli* hedges in the conservation of plant germplasm, should be assessed. When found to be effective such indigenous technologies should be popularised because they are already in the hands of the people.

REFERENCES

Ayensu, E. S. 1983. "Endangered Species used in Traditional Medicine." In *Traditional Medicine and Health Care Coverage: A Reader for Health Administrators and Practitioners* edited by R. H. Bannerman et. al. Geneva: WHO.

Falconer, J. 1990. *The Major Significance of Minor Forest Products*. FAO Community Forestry Note No. 6. Rome: FAO.

FAO. 1986. *Some Medicinal Forest Plants of Africa and Latin America*. Rome: FAO.

Kokwaro, J. O. 1988. "Conservation Status of the Kakamega Forest in Kenya: The Easternmost Relic of the Equatorial Rain Forests of Africa." *Monogr. Syst. Bot. Missouri Bot. Gard*. 25:471-488.

____________. 1976. *Medicinal Plants of East Africa*. Nairobi: East African Literature Bureau.

Morton, J. 1977. *Major Medicinal Species*. Spring Field. Ill: Chan C. Thomas.

Redfern, P. 1992. "Trees Lost Annually. *Daily Nation*," October 6, 1992.

Sindiga, I. 1992. *Ethnomedicine and Health Care in Kenya*. Final Technical Report to the International Development Research Centre. Eldoret: Moi University.

Spencer, P. 1965. *The Samburu: A Study in Gerontocracy in a Nomadic Tribe*. London: Routledge and Kegan Paul.

Swain, T. 1972. *Plants in the Development of Modern Medicine*. Cambridge: Harvard University Press.

Verdcourt, B. and E. C. Trumps. 1969. *Common Poisonous Plants of East Africa*. London: Collins.

Watt, J. M. and M. G. Breyer-Brandwijk. 1962. *Medicinal and Poisonous Plants of Southern and Eastern Africa*. Edinburgh and London: E. and S. Livingstone Ltd.

Chapter 14

DRUG RESEARCH PRIORITIES IN KENYA WITH SPECIAL EMPHASIS ON TRADITIONAL MEDICINE

W.M. Kofi-Tsekpo

Traditional medicines have, for centuries, been used in the management of diseases in man and animals. In recent years the importance of their utilisation in primary health care systems has been emphasised in African as well as other countries. The Government of Kenya has taken a serious step in looking into ways of integrating the use of traditional medicines in the health care systems of the nation. It is therefore necessary to device and adopt methods that would reconcile the use of these medicines in contemporary medical services.

Definitions

Traditional medicines comprise medicaments employed in the practice of traditional medicine; these are usually formulated from materials of plant or animal origin, or inorganic substances, and they may be formulated singly or in combination.

Traditional medicine on the other hand, is the sum total of practices, measures, ingredients and procedures of all kinds, material or otherwise, which from time immemorial had enabled the African to guard against disease, to alleviate his sufferings and cure himself (World Health Organisation, 1978).

Plant-derived medicines

Plant sources have provided the basis for compounds for use in the development of modern pharmaceuticals. Some of these plants are still used with little modification, in their original forms, as had been the case in ancient practices of traditional medicine. Some of such plant-derived medicines are still found as monographs in the current standard pharmacopoeia. A few examples are given below:

1. *Ipecacuanha* B P 1980
   Ipecacuanha consists of the underground organs of *Cephalis ipecacuanha* or of *Cephalis acuminata*. It contains not less than 2.0 per cent of total alkaloids of *ipecacuanha*, calculated as emetine and with reference to the material dried at 100 degrees to 105 degrees.
2. *Prepared Ipecacuanha B P 1980*
   Prepared ipecacuanha is ipecacuanha reduced to a powder not more coarse than a fine powder, adjusted, if necessary, by the addition of powdered lactose or an ipecacuanha powder of lower alkaloidal content, to contain 1.90 to 2.10 per cent of total alkaloids, calculated as emetine and with reference to the material dried at 100 to 105 degrees.
3. The USPA/NF Volume 21 1985 also contains monographs on Ipecacuanha as follows:
   (i) Ipecac
   (ii) Powdered Ipecac
   (iii) Ipecac Syrup

Other plant-derived pharmacopoeia preparations that use the intact drug plant materials are:

4. Hycoscyamus Leaf B P 1980
5. Mastic, B P 1980: A resinous exudation from certain forms of varieties of *Pistacia lentiscus.*
6. Matricaria Flowers, B P 1980: The dried flower-heads of *Matricaria chamomilla.*

The above examples are not intended to justify their importance, but only to show that there are still some traditional preparations which are recognised as useful. It would therefore be desirable to identify our own traditional preparations for integration into our *materia medica*. I would like to propose a method of doing this.

Research Priorities

The complexities of drug research

Drug research is a complex and very expensive affair. It has been estimated that it costs approximately US$320 million to develop a single drug product over a period of 10 to 15 years! Obviously, this kind of money has not been available for the research and development of traditional medicines. What we have tried to achieve at the Kenya Medical Research Institute (KEMRI) is to identify the medicinal potential of some of the traditional medicines. By removing the myth surrounding the traditional doctor, it is easier to view him and his medicines on a modern rational scientific basis and the good practitioners can be separated from the charlatans and masqueraders. This, I believe, we have managed to achieve to a significant degree, and the public is therefore protected not only against being cheated, but also from being given unsafe preparations.

In any drug development process, knowing the chemical entity is one thing, but developing it into a drug product is another. Similarly, knowing a plant as a medicinal plant is very far from knowing how to use it to treat diseases. A single plant extract contains at least one hundred chemical compounds, and it is impossible to know which one is the active substance. Moreover, traditional doctors often use combinations of two or more plant materials in a preparation – sometimes up to 30 or more! That further complicates things. Over the years, the pharmaceutical industry in the developed countries has found it much cheaper to develop drugs through synthesis other than from plants. This means that it would cost much (more than US$ 230 million) to develop a traditional medicine into a drug!

Drug development from traditional medicines

If one could establish the therapeutic usefulness of traditional medicine, then it should be possible to integrate such a medicine in our primary health care systems. Although it may not be possible to pass the traditional medicine through the expensive drug development processes, it should, however, be possible to develop an alternative system based on some of our ancient medical practices. This approach should enable us to take advantage of our time tested alternative medicine, while we look for funds to develop modern type drug products from these medicines. The most important requirements for using traditional medicines in our contemporary society is to establish the identity, safety and efficacy of these medicines.

The essential criteria for medicines

All medicines must satisfy three major criteria for them to be acceptable for use. These are:

(i) identity
(ii) safety
(iii) efficacy.

These criteria have been used to set standards for all drug products including the examples cited above. Conventionally manufactured drugs often meet these criteria and laws are enforced to ensure compliance to them. Such laws, unfortunately, are not readily applicable to traditional medicines. However, it should be possible to devise suitable methods for identity, safety and efficacy that could be applied to such medicines.

Sources of information on traditional medicines

The relevant information on a traditional medicine, either herbal or non-herbal, should include the raw materials used, the method of preparation, and the clinical application. The completeness of this information will determine the usefulness of the medication and will facilitate the setting of standards for their use. This kind of information is referred to as ethnomedical information the availability of which is very vital if proper standards for traditional medicines are to be set for their general application in health care. Such information may be obtained from three sources, namely;

(i) the traditional medical practitioner
(ii) published literature
(iii) oral literature other than the practitioner.

The ethnomedical information from the traditional practitioner could be a very valuable source, but is difficult to obtain due to cultural restrictions. At the same time, published literature is often, at best, incomplete while the validity of the oral literature varies widely and is dependent on the particular source.

The evaluation of a traditional medicine

The evaluation of a traditional medicine can be carried out according to the three criteria mentioned above. Table 14.1 below summarises the strategy for the evaluation of traditional medicines and this approach has been used at KEMRI in the last few years.

Table 14.1: Strategic criteria for evaluation of traditional medicines

Criteria	Ethnomedical information	Additional information
Identity	Clinical data; ethnobotanical data	Formulation data; botanical and chemical information
Efficacy	Clinical information; treatment observation	Standardised trials
Safety	Clinical information	Ethnobotanical-chemical clinical correlations; animal pharmacology and toxicology

This table indicates that a multidisciplinary approach is necessary for the evaluation and standardisation of traditional medicines. It requires integration of ethnobotany, pharmacognosy, phytochemistry, pharmacology and toxicology and other branches of medicine and the pharmaceutical sciences. In the past few years at KEMRI we have applied these disciplines to the evaluation of traditional medicines while we worked closely with some of the experienced traditional doctors. In return for their cooperation these traditional doctors have benefited tremendously from our expertise. They have learnt various methods, techniques and scientific principles that have helped them improve on their practice. Indeed, some of them have become highly successful through interaction with the institute.

The question of priorities

If we must use our traditional medicine that derives from our heritage, what should our priorities be? In my opinion, we should develop methods and systems that will enable us to make full use of these medicines. After scientific methods have been used to establish the safety and efficacy of a traditional medicine, then the laws of the land should provide mechanisms of protecting the people who will use these medicines as well as the practitioners. Suggestions are made below on how this may be achieved.

Legalization of ethnomedical practices

Traditional medicine, or ethnomedicine, is the alternative to allopathic medicine. In its practice, three facets of medicine are combined; clinical medicine, drug manufacture and drug dispensing and administration. Thus, the traditional doctor combines the duties of the clinician, the drug manufacturer, the pharmacist, the nurse and sometimes the midwife. In contemporary medicine, all these health professionals have to be registered practitioners of their trade. They must possess certain minimum qualifications to enable them to practise their respective professions. Furthermore, there are requirements for the manufacture of drug products and the standards they have to meet. In considering the legalization of ethnomedicine and its practice, it is necessary to examine the three facets of medical practice.

Considering the strong cultural elements that are an integral part of ethnomedical practice, it may not be possible to restructure the practice into all three or more facets that currently exist in allopathic medicine. Two legal instruments governing the practice of traditional medicine should be adequate at present. These are: registration of the traditional medical practitioner and the registration of the traditional medicines.

I have outlined below some details on the prerequisites of registering a traditional doctor and his medicines. These are suggestions for consideration:

(i) *Registration of the traditional medical practitioner*

The data required should seek to establish the authenticity of the traditional doctor through his credibility in the community in which he practises. The involvement of the local community worker and the local administration would be desirable (Appendix A).

(ii) *Registration of the traditional medicines*

Due to the complex nature of preparing these medicines, the registration of each medicinal product has to be linked to the practitioner. The following details would be necessary (see Appendix B):

a. particulars of the applicant,
b. identification profiles of the medicine,
c. efficacy profiles,
d. safety profiles
e. botanical, chemical, pharmacological and toxicological evaluations.

Discussion

The Traditional Medicines and Drugs Research Centre of KEMRI has been developing the above approach on the evaluation of traditional medicines since the centre was established in 1985 and it has been proven to be a useful method. Through this approach a number of potentially useful medicines for asthma, malaria, mild hypertension, diabetes, epilepsy, gout and arthritis have been identified for future development. There are others currently under evaluation and whose potentials have not been fully established. Of the six medicines mentioned above, only the medicines for asthma and malaria have been subjected to preliminary human trials. It should be noted that the ethical and legal requirements governing human experimentation are fairly stringent. Therefore, although the traditional doctor has been able to administer these medicines to people freely, the medical staff at the institute are not in a position to do so. Human trial cannot be done until complete information on the medicines has been obtained. At present, many traditional doctors think that by giving us the name of a plant, or by giving us a powder or liquid preparation, we should be able to carry out human trials. But this is not so.

I believe that the lack of legal protection for the traditional doctor and his/her medicines makes him feel insecure in providing complete information on his medicines. I hope that when the traditional doctor has been comprehensively protected, it should be possible to move further in the development and promotion of Kenya's traditional medicines. Until that time comes, it is desirable to find ways of educating the traditional doctors, and the public at large, that KEMRI has not stolen any medicine from the traditional doctors and that with the help of the whole Kenyan public, it has been possible to protect the public from quacks. We have also developed something scientific from our traditions and culture which the scientific world would like to emulate.

Our priorities for the provision of health facilities for our people should be to use all the resources available to us. Those who have acquired specialized knowledge are duty bound to use this gift for the betterment of the people. Traditional medicine has also been defined as *solid amalgamation of modern medical knowhow and ancestral experience*. It behoves us to forge this amalgamation.

REFERENCE

WHO. 1978. *The Promotion and Development of Traditional Medicine*. WHO Technical Report Series 622. Geneva: WHO.

Chapter 15

THE FUTURE OF TRADITIONAL MEDICINE IN AFRICA*

Isaac Sindiga, Mary P. Kanunah, Chacha Nyaigotti-Chacha and Emma S. Mwangola

The foregoing chapters have defined the problem of traditional medicine in Africa. In certain cases, specific recommendations have been put forward. In this chapter we propose to examine the future prospects for traditional medicine in Africa with the use of the Kenyan example under three major headings, namely traditional medicine and health care policy, professionalisation of traditional medicine, and *materia medica* in traditional medicine. We have chosen these three headings because of their applied significance in terms of possible participation of traditional medicine in primary health care. Also, any interventions in traditional medicine are likely to go into these areas.

Traditional Medicine and Health Care Policy

When the WHO recommended the use of traditional medicine in national health

* Some of the ideas weaved in this essay were results of working group discussions at the Lake Bogoria Workshop of 1992. Accordingly we acknowledge the following participants within the respective working groups:

(a) Health policy – Rispah Oduwo, Anne Awori, Joyce Meme, P. K. Ndalut and Emma Mwangola

(b) Professionalisation of traditional medicine – Mary P. Kanunah, E. Agot Kawango, Rosemary Owigar, C. Nyaigotti-Chacha, Francis Kibe, A. G. Gibbe and Isaac Sindiga. The group was later joined by Kofi-Tsekpo, J. A. R. Wembah-Rashid and S. Ogungbemi.

(c) *Materia medica* in traditional medicine – W. M. Kofi-Tsekpo, J.A.R. Wembah-Rashid, Kenneth Jumba, S. Ogungbemi and B. A. Abayo. The detailed report of each working group is available (Sindiga, 1993).

care services (see Chapter 1) it strongly urged cooperation between ethnomedicine and biomedicine. Yet we know from the Kenyan example that both traditional medicine and the modern medicine systems have tended to develop separately; there is little communication between the practitioners of the two systems. At the onset of colonial rule, African traditional medicine in Kenya was suppressed and then ignored. It nonetheless thrived alongside the modern medical system.

As a prerequisite to cooperation between the two systems, there should be detailed understanding of both systems and their contributions to health care at all levels of society. It is, however, clear though that whereas traditional healers recognise biomedicine and refer their patients there, the reverse is not true. One of the reasons for this state of affairs is the perceived and actual competition for clients. There has been little desire within the biomedical establishments–which control health ministries, to support research into traditional medicine. Lack of sufficient funding tells of the scant knowledge that is available on various ethnomedical systems.

In Kenya, there is official government acceptance of traditional medicine. This recognition, given in 1979, was granted partly because of government's inability to spread health care facilities throughout the national territory. Those who have conducted research in the rural areas of the country will attest to the quest for practising licenses by traditional healers. This pursuit for licenses is not based on feelings of illegitimacy by the healers (they are widely respected in their communities) but it arises from the fear of harassment by government agents and the possibility of criminal and/or civil prosecution in case of injury or death to patients and other people.

This dilemma reflects the variance between professed health care policy in which traditional medicine has a place, and government lethargy to operationalise its stated objective. The need for the licensing of traditional healers seeks *inter alia* to obtain legal protection for their practices. The Witchcraft Act of 1975 (revised in 1962 and 1981), which appears as Cap 67 of the Laws of Kenya can be used at any time to stifle legitimate traditional medical practice. Significantly, the Act does not provide for bona fide manufacture, supply or sale of traditional drugs and medicines. Only clear new legislation providing for the practice of traditional medicine would create an environment for the development of traditional medicine. Such legislation, would also provide for the registration and licensing of traditional medicine.

Registration and Licensing of Traditional Healers

Registration involves the "recording of details (age, location, training, experience, etc.) of traditional health practitioners according to their type of practice, in a register which is maintained by an official body" (WHO, 1985:24). Licensing on its part entails: "Formal, written permission from a constituted authority to give traditional health care after meeting stipulated requirements and standards of practice" (WHO, 1985:23).

The demands of registration and licensing are such that a considerable amount of work must be done to verify who is a bona fide traditional healer for purposes of registration. This calls for a professional organization or association to set the minimum required standards for the practice of traditional medicine. We discuss the requirements and obligations of the professionalization of traditional medicine further below.

As already noted, Kenya has no licensing authority for the ethnomedical healers. However, some form of authorisation to practise, especially in urban areas, is obtainable. However, this authorisation, which purports to convey a license, clearly lacks the force of law. Also, it appears that the Ministry of Culture and Social Services registers traditional healers both at the district level and at its headquarters in Nairobi. By October 1990, the Department of Culture in the Ministry had registered 104 individual traditional healers (Personal communication, Director of Culture, October 29, 1990).

Moreover, the Kenya Government has encouraged the formation of traditional healer associations. These associations are also seemingly registered by the Department of Culture. However, the standards an association should meet before registration are not spelt out. The involvement of the Department of Culture in the registration exercise apparently owes to the fact that it is the Department that deals with various cultural aspects of Kenyan life of which traditional medicine is part.

Some traditional medical practitioners, especially in urban areas, obtain trade licenses for their operations. Elsewhere, the provincial administration issues licenses on the payment of a fee. Nyambura Githagui (1985), who studied this aspect, found that in certain districts formal licensing through the offices of the locational chief and the district officer is pervasive. In Kilifi District, for example, healers pay Ksh.500 for a licence; nevertheless there is very strong resentment against paying this large sum of money (Githagui, 1985). Moreover, there are no guidelines with regard to who is to be licensed, in which case it is the chiefs who decide on those to be issued with licenses.

Again, in some districts such as Kilifi, the provincial administration issues permits, especially for purposes of traditional healer travel, and to indicate the presence of a healer in an area (Githagui, 1985). In other cases, healers have letters showing that they have been in contact with government officers about their work. Such letters may not even convey authorisation to practice; however, some traditional healers display them. This appears to be a way of gaining credibility and thus attracting customers (Githagui, 1985).

So far nothing that has been said satisfies registration and licensing requirements in professional categories especially in health care. In the developed countries where health services have remained the monopoly of physicians and a few other professionals, the purpose of licensing appears to be protecting (1) the population against quacks, charlatans and traditional healers with no medical qualifications, and (2) those already established in the medical profession (Stepan, 1985). The import of the second purpose is that biomedical practitioners have always wanted to monopolise the provision of health service partly by setting stringent requirements for the neophytes who wish to join the admission roll.

In the area of traditional medicine, only TBAs appear to have been involved fully in PHC in certain districts. In fact, a national curriculum, together with teaching aids and charts, have been published and launched (Kenya, 1991a; Kenya, 1991b). Whereas we applaud these efforts, it appears that TBAs are made to work as functionaries of the biomedical establishment essentially to reduce the number of cases going to the hospital and making referrals of complicated cases, and are thus likely to lose their status in their communities in the process of incorporation into official health care. Therefore, over the longer term, this arrangement is unsatisfactory. As MacCormack (1986:154) notes,

> They will be at the bottom of the bureaucratic heap, poorly paid or asked to work free, given least prestige, the last to be supplied with drugs and in service training.

In this capacity, TBAs will merely be functioning as some form of extension workers under the Ministry of Health (Last, 1986:3).

Perhaps what is required in this case is collaboration and not incorporation of the two medical systems. *Collaboration* is achieved when the two health sectors make appropriate referrals to one another on a routine basis. In the process, certain traditional healing skills are upgraded while at the same time increasing the cultural sensitivity of biomedical workers (Green and Makhubu, 1984:1077).

An operational policy should be formulated that also involves other cadres of traditional medical workers in PHC. Such policy would need to be implemented, monitored and evaluated within the national health care programme. However, a community based programme for practising traditional medicine appears to be the only way to proceed. Eventually an all-encompassing curriculum incorporating the various practices within traditional medicine in the country must be worked out. Such curriculum could form an integral part in the training of various health cadres to sensitise them about traditional medicine.

Professionalization of Traditional Medicine

With government encouragement, associations of traditional healers have been formed in Kenya (Kenya, 1989:224). Such include *Umoja wa Waganga wa Mitishamba* and Association of African Traditional Medical Practitioners of Kenya. It appears that the role of these associations is to foster traditional medicine in order to complement official health services. In the words of the 1989-1993 National Development Plan, these associations:

> will facilitate the gathering of necessary information for the use, development and appropriate adaptation of traditional diagnostic, therapeutic and rehabilitative control technologies that will become part and parcel of formal medical research and of the Primary Health Care Programme (Kenya, 1989:244).

But the question whether these associations may be considered professional is another matter altogether. All the same, it is clear that the government's intention is to make these associations professional.

A profession is a constituted occupation which has some degree of independence, keeps a monopoly over a defined sphere of work, contains a code of ethics, and is brought together by a body of knowledge and skills which it holds on behalf of and in service to society (Last, 1986:6). It follows that a profession regulates its members, retains control over licensing, enforces its regulations, and participates in the teaching and examination of recruits and in promoting research (Last, 1986:6-7). It is the specialised knowledge which a group of people has, according to Last, which becomes the source of authority of a given profession. Thus, organising into a professional group or association provides legitimacy to the people so doing (MacCormack, 1986).

The urge to professionalize must be tempered with meeting certain standards expected of a professional body – obtaining an examinable uniform standard, testing the efficacy and safety of treatments and attaining uniform quality of care, all of which require institutional initiation through training (Last, 1986; Chapter 3). Table 15.1 shows some characteristics of allopathic medicine including training together with those of ethnomedicine.

African traditional medicine is part of the culture in which it exists. This means that traditional medical practice complies with the social set-up and cultural etiquette of the society. A myriad socio-cultural changes are taking place in Africa thereby removing whatever controls existed over traditional medicine. According to Green and Makhubu (1984), the spur to form ethnomedical healer associations is the desire to enforce discipline on healers and distance themselves from charlatans, ritual murderers and quacks. Thus, a healers' association should

Table 15.1: Major characteristics of allopathic and ethnomedical practices

Allopathic	Ethnomedical
Western	**Indigenous**
— Universally accepted and globally spread, cosmopolitan.	— Existence universally accepted but practice is regionalised and culture-specific although it may traverse cultural boundaries. No absolute cultural uniformity.
— Training is rigorous and takes specified period of time. Sealed by certification and registration	— Training process and period vary from one practitioner and area of specialisation to another. May be sealed with symbolic amulets, dressing etc.
— Hierarchy of resort in both human and physical facilities – i.e. referrals to specialists of different levels and to experience and to different grades of health institutions.	— Hierarchy of resort in personnel. Referrals among practitioners limited due to commercialisation of the "profession", plus jealousy.
— Institutionalised – buildings, wards, theatres, morgues, laboratories, consulting rooms, drugs, equipment (permanent and consumable)	— Homes may serve as health centres; practitioners may visit a patient at his/her home or at the home of therapy managing group member.
— Personnel categorised: doctors, nurses, clinicians, laboratory technicians, physiotherapists, pharmacists, technologists, etc.	— Often an individual's show; occasionally with relatives or apprentices to run errands and learn on the job.
— Trainees must meet certain qualification for admission.	— Certain characteristics required but not mandatory.
— Use of special equipment/tools of the profession.	— Special healers have special instruments; e.g. bone-setters, surgeons, diviners, etc.
— Procedures of diagnoses: case history, physical examination, laboratory test and X-ray.	— Physical examination; usually oral case history; hardly specimen tests; 'X-rays' by use of mirror, water, bible, lamp, etc.
— Health management process compartmentalised; with the consultant different from the drug manufacturer and also from drug dispenser and administrator	— In its practice, the three facets of medicine-clinical medicine, drug manufacture and drug dispensing and administration, are combined and wrapped up in one person, the healer.
— Medicines and drugs are developed in stages and experimented on different animals before being used on humans. (Takes years to be accepted).	— Medicines and drugs are developed over many years through trial and error and familiarity with the environment. Some claims to inspirational sources entertained.

SOURCE: *Traditional Medicine: Its Practice and the Law in Kenya* edited by I. Sindiga (1993).

promote traditional medicine through registration, fees regulation and drawing up a code of conduct (Green and Makhubu, 1984).

Sindiga's (1992) study among the Luo and Maasai shows that healers in rural areas are not members of any healer association; they work quietly in their areas as they have done for centuries. However, the situation is different for urban healers who seek to protect themselves and obtain legitimacy through membership of an association (Last, 1986). However, the objectives of Kenya's traditional healer associations are not well known. We recommend research in this area to provide data for further comment on their suitability to act as professional associations.

It is clear that Kenya's urban traditional healers would like to survive by attracting clients through appealing invitations — the use of such titles as "doctor" and even "professor" is now a common feature among them. Yet these titles are not given by any organisation; individual healers just "award" themselves and use them. Since these titles are normally earned on the attainment of certain standards in formal training, their liberal use by traditional medical practitioners only tells of their craving for public rather than professional recognition.

We believe that traditional medicine requires some form of regulation. It is not clear how traditional healer associations will do this but their existence is helpful in sorting out what is useful in traditional medicine and what is not. The associations should inculcate a spirit of professionalism and a sense of responsibility to society by their members rather than acting merely as trade unions for self-defence and self-preservation.

Materia Medica in Traditional Medicine

Every medical system has its own drugs and other pharmacopoeia and hence the necessity to study *materia medica* in traditional medicine. The term *materia medica* (or ingredients of the medicines) refers to a compilation of monographs of medicines for different diseases. Each monograph represents a given medication and specifies the name, the raw materials used to prepare the medicine, method of preparation, use, mode of administration, dose, and other relevant data such as contraindications and storage.

The proposals for a Kenyan *materia medica* with regard to traditional medicine is justified on the premise that it would provide data for new drug development. This *materia medica* would be an invaluable documentation of the cultural and traditional treatments among different ethnic groups and in different geographical locations of the country (C.f Chapter 12). The urgency of compiling a Kenyan *materia medica* is that the elders, who are the repositories of such information are slowly dying. Medicinal herbs are being destroyed as well. This is a challenge to researchers. However this task requires a multi-disciplinary team of experts dedicated to the research.

Concluding Remark

Throughout the world indigenous knowledge systems are being "rediscovered". This has come about as a result of dissatisfaction with advanced technologies which are, nonetheless, impractial and unsustainable because of environmental and cultural insensitivity. This is the case with indigenous systems of medicine.

To foster traditional medicine in Africa, interventions are required in the three areas which have been outlined in this chapter, namely health policy, professionalisation and materia medica. Concrete steps should be taken to do the task beginning with the creation of an enabling environment within which traditional medicine can flourish. We owe it to posterity.

REFERENCES

Githagui, N. 1985. *Traditional Healing Practices in Kenya: A Study of Four Kenyan Communities*. Nairobi. AMREF.

Green, E. C. and L. Makhubu. 1984. "Traditional Healers in Swaziland: Toward Improved Cooperation Between the Traditional and Modern Sectors" *Social Science and Medicine* 18 No. 12: 1071-1079.

Kenya, Government of. 1989. *Development Plan 1989-1993*. Nairobi: Government Printer.

_______. 1991a. *National Curriculum for Traditional Birth Attendants*. Nairobi: Ministry of Health in Conjunction with WHO and the Government of Belgium.

_______. 1991b. *Traditional Birth Attendants Trainers Guide*. Nairobi: Ministry of Health and WHO Kenya Office.

Last, M. 1986. "The Professionalisation of African Medicine: Ambiguities and Definitions" In *The Professionalisation of African Medicine* edited by M. Last and G. L. Chavunduka. Manchester: Manchester University Press. pp. 1-19.

MacCormack, C. 1986. "The Articulation of Western and Traditional Systems of Health Care." In *The Professionalisation of African Medicine* edited by M. Last and G. L. Chavunduka. Manchester: Manchester University Press. pp. 151-162.

Sindiga, I. 1992. *Ethnomedicine and Health Care in Kenya*. Final Technical Report to the International Development Research Centre. Eldoret: Moi University.

Sindiga, I. (ed). 1993. *Traditional Medicine, Its Practice and the Law in Kenya*. Proceedings of the National Workshop, Lake Bogoria Hotel, 4-7 November, 1992. Eldoret: Moi University.

Stepan, J. 1985. "Traditional and Alternative Systems of Medicine: A Comparative Review of Legislation" *International Digest of Legislation* 36 No. 2:283-341.

WHO. 1985. *Report of the Consultation on Approaches for Policy Development for Traditional Health Practitioners Including Traditional Birth Attendants*. Geneva: WHO.

APPENDIX A

APPLICATION FOR THE REGISTRATION OF TRADITIONAL MEDICAL PRACTITIONERS

REGISTRATION SERIAL NO..................
(for official use only)

1. Name of Applicant (Last Name) ____________________

   (Other Names) ____________________

2. Postal Address ____________________

3. Business Address ____________________

4. National Identification No. ____________________

5. Age ____________________

6. Place of Birth ____________________

7. Number of Years in Practice ____________________

8. Give a brief account of training experience ____________________

9. State your areas of specialisation ____________________

10. State the last two places you stayed before coming to the present address:

    (i) Location/Town ____________________

    Period of stay ______________ 19______ to ______________ 19 ______

    Occupation during this period ____________________

    (ii) Location/Town

    Period of stay ______________ 19______ to ______________ 19 ______

11. Certification by the District Officer at the present address:

I certify that (Name)______________________________ is a traditional practitioner/midwife and has been resident in this location during the last_______ years/months.

Name of District Officer ____

Signature _______________________ Date __________________________

12. Certification by the District Commissioner at the present address:

I certify that (Name)____

has been acknowledged by the people in this district as a genuine traditional practitioner/midwife.

Name of District Commissioner ______________________________________

Signature _______________________ Date __________________________

13. I certify that the information given in this application form is, to my best knowledge, correct.

Signature of Applicant ____

Date ____

APPENDIX B

APPLICATION FORM FOR THE REGISTRATION OF TRADITIONAL MEDICINES

REGISTRATION SERIAL NO..................
(for official use only)

PROPOSED NAME OF THE TRADITIONAL MEDICINE ____________________

____

PART A

PARTICULARS OF THE APPLICANT

1. Applicant's names: Last Name____________________

   Other Names____________________

2. National Identification Number____________________

3. Postal Address____________________

4. Business Address____________________

5. State briefly the extent of your experience____________________

   ____

   ____

6. How many business locations do you operate at? Give the addresses

   ____

   ____

7. I certify that the information given in all sections of this application form is, to the best of my knowledge, correct. I have given the information in strict confidence, with the understanding that it will be used for registration purposes only.

______________________________ ______________________

Signature Date

PART B

IDENTIFICATION PROFILES OF THE MEDICINE

1. **Raw Materials:**

How many plants are used in the preparation of the medicine? _______________

Give below the botanical names with local language name equivalents.

Plant Name	Local Name	Parts used (state whether fresh or dried)
1.		
2.		
3.		
4.		
5.		
6.		

(b) Are any other plants or materials used in the preparation of this medicine?

Yes/No____

If yes, give details____

2. **Preparation of the Medicine:**

(a) Describe concisely how the medicine is prepared from the above-named materials:____

____

____

(b) Is the medicine given to the patient in the powdered/solid form?

Yes/No____

If Yes, state clearly the instructions to be given for preparation and administration

____

____

____

(c) Is the medicine to be given to the patient in liquid form?

Yes/No ____

If Yes, state clearly the instructions for administration____________________

____

____

(d) How long will the preparation last before it becomes unusable?

For the powder/solid____

For the liquid ____

____

(e) Note: Samples of the medicine should be submitted with the application form.

PART C

EFFICACY PROFILES

Ethnomedical applications

1. What is the major indication of the medicine?______________________________

____

2. Other indication (if any)____

____

3. State the approximate period of medication______________________________

____

PART D

SAFETY PROFILES

1. What side effects can be observed on excessive or prolonged use of this medicine?____

____

2. What are the contraindications?____

____

PART E

(For Official Use Only)

BOTANICAL, CHEMICAL, PHARMACOLOGY AND TOXICOLOGICAL EVALUATIONS

1. Have plants belonging to any of the following botanical classes been mentioned in Part B of this form?

(i) Boraginacea - all genera
(ii) Compositae – tribes: (a) Senecioneae
(b) Eupatoriae
(iii) Leguminosae – Genus: Crotalaria

If Yes, name them____

____

2. Has the absence of pyrrolizidine alkaloids and mycotoxins been proven in the preparation? Yes/No.

3. What is the level of microbial contamination? __________________________

____

4. Has any peculiar pharmacological activity been identified in the medicinal preparation? Yes/No. If Yes, describe briefly__________________________

____

5. What is the published literature information on the medicinal plants used in this medicinal preparation? Give a brief account with copies of the publications where possible____

____

6. Recommendation of the Technical Evaluation Committee

____

____

____

__________________________ __________________________

Signature of Chairman Date

INDEX

A

Abagusii 33, 108-114
  disease aetiology 109
  traditional medicine 109-11
  witchcraft 109-111
Abaluyia 117-128
  disease aetiology 117
  taboos 119-120
  traditional medicine 124-128
Abrus precatorius 148
Abrus schimperi 148
Acacia brevispica 148
Acacia gerrardii 148
Acacia nilotica 95
Acacia seyal 95
Acanthus sp 159
Achyranthus aspera 160, 161
Acocanthera longifolia 147
Acocanthera schimperi 147
Aconitum 144
Aconitum napellus 144
acupuncture 3, 22, 44, 64
Adenium obesum 147
Adenium somalonse 147
Afzelia quanzensis 162
Ageratum conyzoides 157
Aids 4, 35, 48, 49, 63, 68
Albizia anthelminthica 95
Albizia coriara 163
ALDEV 156
Alma Ata International Conference 3, 4
Alstonia boonei 159, 163
Amaranthus hybridus 132
AMREF 85
Apocyanaceae 146, 147-148
Aristolochia sp 142
Artemisia afra 159, 160
Asia 1, 4, 143
Association of African Traditional Medical
Practitioners of Kenya 179
asthma 110, 114, 146, 173
Atropa belladona 144
ayurveda 3, 44, 50, 64, 142
Azadirachta indica 159, 163

B

bilharzia 133
biomedicine 18, 19, 22, 24, 25, 32, 41, 42-43, 44, 45, 50, 51, 84, 90, 105 (see also medicine, modern)
Bischoffia javanica 162
Blighia unjuguta 164
Boscia salicifolia 161
Bridelia micrantha 163
bubonic plague 121
Bungoma 117
Busia 117, 159, 160

C

Caesalpinia volkensii 164
Cajanus cajan 149
Calotrophis procera 160
cancer 35
Cannabis sativa 144
Capparis erythrocarpos 160, 161, 165
Carissa edulis 148, 160
Cassia sp 95, 148
Cassia abbreviata 148
Cassia didymobotrya 148, 160
Cassia floribuda 148
Cassia mimosoides 148
Cassia occidentalis 148, 160
Cassia senna 148
Cassia siamea 163, 164
Cassia singuena 148
Catharathus roseus 147
Cephalis ipecacuanha 169
chemotherapy 56
China 3, 4, 44, 49, 141, 145
chiropractic 3, 22, 44, 50

Chlorophora exelsa 160, 162, 163, 164
cholera 1
CIKARD 19
CIRAN 19
Cinchona cordifolia 144
Cinchona ledgeriana 144
Cinchona officianalis 144
circumcision 98, 113, 138
Cissus quadrangularis 96
Claviceps purpurea 144, 145
Commiphora africana 163
Congo 160
Cordia africa 162
Croton onacrostachyus 132
Croton zambesieus 95
Culture and Social Services, Ministry of 177

D

Dalbergia melanoxylon 162
Datura stramonium 50, 144, 146
Datura metel 146
Delonix ragia 164
Desauax-Holarrhena pubescens 147
diarrhoea 20, 65, 66, 86, 89, 111, 148, 157
diabetes 144
Dichrostachys cinerea 148
Digitalis purpurea 144, 147
disease (**see also illness**) 1, 18, 19-20, 21, 22, 31-32, 40, 65-68, 80-81, 87-91, 109-111, 117-124, 125, 130, 131
    aetiology 9, 18, 20, 32, 64, 65-68, 82-83, 109-111, 117-124, 125, 130, 131
    dichotomy 33-34
dysentery 1, 86, 148

E

Ekebergia rueppelliana 159, 162
Embella kilimandscharica 95
Entada abyssinia 149, 160
Ephedra sp 145
Erythrina abyssinia 132, 161, 164
Erythrophlem africanum 148
ethics 35, 136, 179-181
ethnomedicine (**see also traditional medicine**) 3, 9, 16-18, 19, 58-63, 84, 85, 154, 172
    definition 18, 19-20
    practice 55-63
eucalyptus 164, 166

F

Fagara macrophylla 157, 159, 160, 162

G

Gardenia lutea 163
Githae, Jack 50
gonorrhoea 114, 133, 148
Grevilla robusta 164

H

Hagenia abyssinia 162
health 18, 31, 80-81, 133
    definition 20
Health, Ministry of 63, 178
Helleborus niger 144
herbal medicines; (**see medicinal plants**)
herbal therapy 31, 32, 40, 41-42, 57, 61-62, 68-78, 83, 86, 87, 89-90, 91, 110, 114, 115, 140-149
herbalists; (**see traditional healers**)
Hippocrates 56
Holarrhena febrifuga 147
Homa Bay 70, 155
homeopathy 3, 22, 44, 50, 142
Hyosyamus niger 144

I

illness (**see also disease**) 18, 31, 32
immunization 2, 34, 46, 88, 133
India 4, 44, 49, 50, 145
Institute of Alternative Medicine and

Technology 50

J

Jateorhiza palmata 159
Jatropha curcas 164

K

Kajiado 95
Kakamega 117, 119, 159, 160, 161, 163
Kamba 33, 40, 42
Karati Rural service Centre (KRSC) 55, 57-63
KEFRI 154
Keiyo 23
KEMRI 7, 11, 169, 172, 173, 174
Kenya 5-8, 30, 31, 33, 36-37, 38, 41, 44, 45, 46, 48, 51, 55-63, 64, 65, 88, 118, 129, 140, 141, 143, 145-149, 175, 176
Kenyatta National Hospital 63
Kericho 57, 159
Khaya senegalensis 159, 162
Kikuyu 10-11, 33, 129-139
    disease aetiology 133-134
    medicineman 134-136
    traditional medicine 129-139
    witchcraft 133
Kilifi 177
Kinangop 57, 58
Kisii 113, 155, 156
Kisumu 65, 155, 159, 160, 161, 164
Kuria 33, 113

L

laibon 97-100
Lannea stuhlmanni 163
LEAD 19
Leucaena leucocephala 149
Leguminoceae 146, 148-149
Leonotis sp 157
Leprosy 121, 122
Luo 9-10, 20, 23, 64-78, 80-91, 157, 161, 181
Lycium europaeum 147

M

Maasai 10, 20, 94, 95-106, 181
    disease aetiology 101-102
    traditional healers 97-100, 102-106
    traditional medicine 94-97
    witchcraft 101-102
Maba 95
Machakos 44, 161
Maesa lanciolata 96
Maeura edulis 160, 161, 165
magic 17, 49, 130 (**see also witchcraft**)
Makini, Morris 47-49, 50
malaria 1, 65, 66, 86, 111, 148, 173
Mandrax officinarum 144
Marakwet 23, 133
materia medica 12, 175, 181-182
Matricaria chamomilla 169
measles 65, 87, 132, 151
medical pluralism 16, 23-24, 64
medical systems 9, 16-26, 64
    definitions 17
medicinal plants 31, 49, 55-57, 94-97, 141-151, 153-166, 168, 169-174
    advantages of 55-56
    research 60-61, 62, 66, 166, 169-174
    sources 59-60, 157, 158
    trade in 155, 158-159
medicine, modern (**see also biomedicine**) 1, 4-6, 18-19, 22, 24, 25-26, 32, 36, 37, 38, 39, 41, 42-43, 44, 45, 46, 50, 51, 55, 84, 90, 105
medicineman (**see traditional healer**)
Meru 133
Mitragyana stipulosa 159, 163
Mohammed, Shariff Omar 49
Moi University 45
Morbidity 1

mortality rates 1, 2, 4, 65, 86
Murang'a 129
Myrica kilimanshuarica 96

N

Nairobi 5, 7, 47, 57, 94, 143
Naivasha 57
Narium oleander 147
Narok 95, 102, 103, 106, 161
Nyahururu 57
Nyamira 156
Nyandarua 57, 129
Nyanza 6, 86, 87, 88, 153, 166, 159
Nyeri 57, 129

O

Occium basilicum 160, 161
Ocotea usambarensis 159, 162
Olea welwistschii 162
ormocarpum trichocarpum 161

P

Paeonia sp 141
Papppea capensis 95, 160
Pappea guinensis 159, 160
Papaver somnifera 141, 144
Penicillin 144
Piliostigma thonningii 149
Pistacia lentiscus 169
Plumbago zeylanica 164
Podocarpus gracilior 162
Podocarpus milanjianus 162
Pokot 33
Primary health Care 1, 2, 3-5, 18, 25-26, 30, 31, 35, 36-39, 80-81, 133, 175-178
Prunus africanum 162
psychotherapy 133

R

Raowolfia caffa 147, 159
Raowalfia mombasiana 147
Raowolfia serpenfica 145, 147
Raowolfia vomitoria 147, 160
religion 44-45, 78, 102, 124-125, 126-127, 130, 136-137
rheumatism 20, 145
Rhoicissus eythrodes 95
Ricinus communis 141, 146
Rift Valley 6, 87
ringworm 86
roundworm 86

S

Sclerocarya birrea 159, 163
schistosomiasis 1, 65
Siaya 45, 65, 81, 155
skin diseases 20, 65, 85, 121
small pox 121, 132
Solanaceae 146
Solanum aculeastrum 146
Solanum dasyphyllum 146
Solanum goetzel 146
Solanum incanum 146, 160, 161
Solanum nigrium 146
sorcery (**see witchcraft**)
South Nyanza 5, 64-78
spirits 120-121, 125, 130-132
Steganotaenia araliacea 161, 165
Strophanthus emini 147
Strophanthus kombo 147
Strychnos henningsii 133
Strychnos nux-vomica 144, 145
syphillis 147, 148

T

taboos 80, 82, 83, 119-120, 122, 125, 130, 161
Tamarindus indica 148
Tanzania 9, 21, 47, 94
Teclea noblis 160
Tecona stans 160, 164
therapy-seeking behaviour 9, 68-78, 111, 121-124
Thevetia peruviana 147, 164
Thika 129

Tilthonia diversifolia 164
Toddalia asatica 157
traditional birth attendants 32, 35, 84, 91, 124, 126, 138, 178
traditional healers 3, 4, 7, 16-17, 20, 22, 32-35, 41-50, 51, 56, 66-70, 89-90, 97, 102-106, 111-115, 127, 134-136, 137, 138, 143, 155, 157, 159, 160, 163, 164, 176-178
    associations 177, 179-181
    categories 21, 32, 67-70, 112, 135
    research 62-63
    urban 48, 49, 50, 139, 181
traditional medicine 1, 3, 4-5, 7, 19, 23-26, 30-39, 40-53, 55-63, 80-91, 94-106, 124-128, 129-139, 140-151, 153-166, 168-174, 175-181
    constraints 25, 34-35
    definition 19-20, 168-169
    ethics 35, 136, 179-181
    integration of 24-25, 36-39
    legislation 34, 37-38, 52, 63, 172-170, 176-178
    research 26, 35, 62
Traditional Medicines and Drugs Research Centre 173
Traditional Medicines Unit 7
Trichillia emetica 162
trypanosomiasis 1
tuberculosis 1
Turkana 5-6
typhoid 1

U

Uganda 49, 65, 159
urginea sp 141
UNICEF 2, 85
University of Nairobi 7, 63

V

Valeriana officinalia 142
Vihiga 117, 119

W

Warbugia ugandensis 159, 161, 163
Witchcraft Act 34, 136, 176
witchcraft 16-17, 20 24, 25, 34, 40, 51-52, 57, 66-67, 101-102, 109, 113, 117-119, 122-123, 125, 133, 136-137
witchdoctor 16-17, 40, 31, 32, 52, 142
Withania somnifera 146
World health Assembly 3-4
World Health Organisation 1, 2, 3, 24, 88, 175

Z

Zaire 77
Zambia 4
Zanthoxylum usambarense 157
Zaramo 9, 21
Zimbabwe 4